THE ANOINTING TO HEAL

THE ANOINTING TO HEAL

Randolph Vickers

Terra Nova Publications

Reprinted in 2006

Published in Great Britain by
Terra Nova Publications International Ltd
PO Box 2400, Bradford on Avon, Wiltshire BA15 2YN

Registered Office (not for trade):
21 St Thomas Street, Bristol BS1 6JS

Cover design by Roger Judd

ISBN 1 901949 38 9

Printed in Great Britain
by Bookmarque Ltd, Croydon

Contents

PREFACE

In 1991 The Northumbrian Centre of Prayer for Christian Healing was established at our home to be a safe place for people to come and meet with the only one we can fully trust, our Lord Jesus. He is the one who can bring us into true healing and wholeness. Although we did not realize it when we bought the house, its name, 'Beggars Roost', has very special significance. A beggar is someone who is beyond his own resources —like those who are sick and are seeking healing. There are so many people today who are in need of healing and many who are desolate, lonely, with no hope, no opportunities, nowhere to go, no-one they feel they can trust. They certainly cannot trust themselves.

The theme of God sheltering his children as they encounter the storms of life is one that has been with me for many years. I am reminded of the precious words of Psalm 91:4, the truth of which we have seen for ourselves on so many occasions, both here and elsewhere:

He will cover you with his feathers,
and under his wings you will find refuge;
his faithfulness will be your shield and rampart.

This book tells some of the story of how, in the years since 1975, when Jesus began to involve my wife Dorothy and myself in his ministry of healing, people have come and we have gone out – to many other places in the UK and overseas – and we have seen Jesus heal.

Although this book recounts the stories of many who were healed through the outreach of the Centre, it is not intended to be triumphalist. Whilst many stories of those who received healing are recorded here, there are others, including members of our team, who have not yet manifested their healing, so we readily acknowledge that we live within that tension. It is hoped that *The Anointing to Heal* will provide encouragement and be a source of useful information for churches, groups and individuals working with Jesus in his ministry of healing, or thinking about getting involved. We also trust that, through these accounts of healing, those who are sick, and their friends and families, will grow in hope and trust that with our Father God all things are possible.

Using as examples only the details of some of the healings I have personally witnessed (in order that I can vouch for their authenticity) I have tried to demonstrate some of the ways in which we actually go about the ministry. In many cases I describe what we do and why we do it, what we say and why we say it, wherever possible providing the scriptural basis for our actions.

When, at one stage, I contemplated scrapping any idea of writing a book, I was phoned early one morning by a lady whom I had not seen or heard of for more than a year. The Lord had impressed on her to telephone me with this verse: *"Is not my word like fire,"* *declares the LORD, "and like a hammer that breaks a rock in pieces?"* (Jeremiah 23:29). She said that I probably did not realise the impact this healing Centre had had on people all over the place, and the number of healings, both mental and physical, which had been received through our work, nor that so many ministries and groups had risen from the ministry and teaching we had conducted elsewhere. She told me how, some years earlier, she had come to Beggars Roost, where she was released from fear. Now she and her husband are in ministry themselves.

This book is dedicated to Dorothy as we have worked together in this ministry for thirty years; to the team at The Northumbrian Centre of Prayer for Christian Healing, which is now under the direction of our son David and his wife Karen, who have made it possible for us to travel extensively over the years; also to all those ministers who have welcomed us into their churches. I especially want to thank Dorothy, and our friend Nora Scott, for proof reading, and Ellen Mallay for seeking out permission to use people's names and stories.

Randolph Vickers
Beggars Roost
August 2005

1

A FUNNEL OF GOD'S LOVE
FOR HEALING

The Lord showed me that I was to be a 'funnel' of his love. That is the picture he gave to me of the Christian's role in Jesus' ministry of healing: a funnel through which he can pour his love, peace, grace and healing power into those who need him.

I suppose that I possibly got the first glimpse of this when my wife Dorothy and I were ministering in East Germany, before the wall came down. We did not speak any German. Our host, guide and interpreter was my friend Jean Pierre Witzman, the Berlin President of the Full Gospel Businessmens' Fellowship International (FGBMFI). After worship and my talk, we came to a time for ministry. Jean Pierre announced in German that anyone who required prayer should come forward. It was a small room, packed with people. Some space was made in the front. A little elderly lady shuffled forward; all her joints were stiff, and she moved with difficulty. She spoke no English and Jean Pierre was occupied with other people. So I simply laid hands on her by gently holding her shoulders. The Lord showed me how cold and desolate she was inside, not physically cold because of the temperature of the room, but emotionally and spiritually frozen. It felt like a cold, devastated wasteland inside of her, with no hope. I was filled with the understanding that all she had loved and cared for had been taken away from her. I asked Dorothy to hold her. Dorothy is only 5 feet 2 inches, but she was considerably taller than this little woman, and was able to wrap her arms around the lady and cuddle her. We prayed silently in tongues. Dorothy held her for what seemed a very long time until she felt that the Lord had done all that was necessary. As Dorothy held the lady, Father God poured love and warmth and hope and peace, and who knows what more, into her very being, quickening and releasing her imprisoned spirit. All that was required of us was to be there and be willing to be his arms so that he could love her back to life. By twisting and wriggling our bodies we demonstrated that we wanted her to wriggle and move. As she wriggled, she realised that the love of God had brought warmth and healing into the frozen wasteland within her; that her very joints and bones had been unfrozen, and she had been set free. When she went back to her place in the congregation she did not shuffle but walked freely. One of the lasting impressions in my mind was of what took place after the meeting had finished and everyone was leaving. The little lady, whose name we never even knew, turned her head when she got to the door, looked over her shoulder, smiled at us with a merry twinkle in her eye and then cheekily wiggled her bottom at us, to show she was healed and free. I was reminded of Malachi 4:2, *But for you who revere my name, the sun of righteousness will rise with healing in its wings. And you will go out and leap like calves released from the stall.* That little, round, elderly lady literally skipped out of the room. In retrospect, I realised that this was the first glimmerings of what many years later I was to call 'absorption theology'. I realised that the great gift that we can bring to people is the overwhelming presence of God's love in the power of the Holy Spirit. Healing comes through soaking in the anointing of the Holy Spirit so that we simply absorb into our very being the healing love of Jesus, without needing to be consciously aware or our brain necessarily having any understanding of what is happening. Healing is absorbing into our total being – spirit, soul and body – the wholeness that is from Christ Jesus. Ephesians 1:3f teaches us that Father God has blessed us in the heavenly realms with every spiritual blessing in Christ. Jesus wants to pour blessings into us.

I cannot heal anyone. Although God has given our bodies the natural ability to heal, we cannot consciously heal ourselves. It is the will of God to heal, and he does the healing. We soak in him and absorb it. So in ministering to people, as our arms go round them, somehow we bring them into the presence of Christ. Our arms become the opening of the funnel into them, through which he lavishes upon them the riches of his grace. (See Ephesians 1:7)

Part of the vision the Lord gave me for setting up the Northumbrian Centre of Prayer for Christian Healing here in Beggars Roost was to teach and encourage the body of Christ at large to embrace his ministry of healing. This would entail going out to other churches and congregations, both here and overseas, as we were invited. Therefore I had to know why churches and congregations were not actively involved in healing. I found that fear is the predominant problem, and poor teaching on faith and belief, and the relationship between them, compounds this.

The fear voiced, both by ministers and their congregations, is: 'But what about the ones who don't get healed?' It appears to them that to accept a theology for healing means accepting a God who is partial, in that he will heal some and not others, whereas the Scriptures tell us that God is impartial.

Then Peter began to speak: "I now realize how true it is that God does not show favoritism" (Acts 10:34).

'For God does not show favoritism' (Romans 2:11)
The truth of the Scriptures can appear to contradict the experience of the churches. Therefore they probably feel that it is safer not to get involved with divine healing in the first place. Is it not strange that people do not have the same problem in relation to secular medicine? The evidence is that many people who undergo medical treatment do not get well, and many die, but no one suggests that we should therefore stop going to consult the physician. Maybe the difference for them between medical healing and divine healing is that with the former they do not feel at fault if they do not get well.

Return for a moment to the issue of fear. On the part of those who are sick, there can be fear that if they go forward for prayer and do not get healed it might be their fault. Did they not have enough faith to be healed? How will it look in the eyes of others? Ministers may be fearful that, if they lay hands on the sick and they do not get well, it might mean that he (the minister) does not have sufficient faith. Therefore it can feel safer for the sick person to sit in the pew and cope with the problem; to stay sick and not take the chance. It can feel safer from the minister's point of view not to invite the sick to come forward for laying on of hands for healing. To invite people to come forward for a blessing is safer, because that could mean all kinds of things which are not necessarily immediately observable. Neither

11

the minister nor the sick person can feel at fault with a blessing.

There are probably as many theologies of healing as there are theologians, and I have discussed many of them in greater depth in my MA thesis 'Aspects of Healing'. It may seem superfluous or even presumptuous to name another one, 'absorption theology', but in none of the others can I find the concept of the osmosis type of process which I perceive divine healing to be.

Although we are involved in ministering with the expectation that we will see the manifestation of the healing as we speak to the problem, there should be no fear on the part of the supplicant or the ministry team, because I believe that healing is a process not an event. Even when there is the evidence and experience of an instantaneous physical healing, or relief from mental anguish, during prayer or through the laying on of hands, this is just an instant in the whole process of preparation that has been going on in the life of that person. This process has also been going on in the life of the person who is ministering, and in the lives of any others included, such as those witnessing the healing. For instance, the friends who lowered the paralytic through the roof, so that Jesus could heal him, were very much involved in the preparation and the whole process of the healing.

When I accepted Jesus as Lord in my life I acknowledged my own participation in this journey of appreciation and understanding of wholeness. I believe that God has already provided all that we need, and that it is his will both that his people may prosper in all respects, as their soul prospers, and that they enjoy good health. We need to come into a place of acceptance and being able to receive. Wrestling with the question of how do we come into the place to receive (or appropriate) what is his will for us, I realised both how essential, how central, is the emphasis that Jesus places on the kingdom of heaven being at hand, and that healing now is only possible because the kingdom of God is here now. When Jesus (in Luke 9:1f) gives the twelve power and authority, he instructs them to do two things: firstly to proclaim the kingdom of God, and secondly to perform healing. Then with the seventy: *Heal the sick who are there and tell them, 'The kingdom of God is near you'* (Luke 10:9). And, *From that time on Jesus began to preach, "Repent, for the kingdom of heaven is near."* (Matthew 4:17). [Many versions (including AV) translate the word *eggizo* here as 'at hand' rather than 'near'.]

Jesus went throughout Galilee, teaching in their synagogues, preaching the good news of the kingdom, and healing every disease and sickness among the people (Matthew 4:23).

"The time has come," he said. "The kingdom of God is near. Repent and believe the good news!" (Mark 1:15).

Here, too, other versions say the kingdom of God is at hand. Thus the good news of the kingdom is central to Jesus' teaching and ministry. He was not just talking about a kingdom that was to come sometime in the future, part of our future hope, a purely eschatological experience in which we will also be made whole and released from all sickness and disease. No, this was and is for the present moment.

What would I do if, say, I decide to bake a cake? I would check that I had all the ingredients and lay them out on the kitchen counter. I would get out the utensils needed: the spoons, the whisk, cake tins. When they were all assembled in a convenient place I would start to mix the cake. I would not start until everything was at hand, so I could just reach out and pick what I need, as I required; there need be no running around frantically, wondering do I have this or that ingredient and trying to remember where I had possibly put the egg whisk last time I used it. Everything would be at hand.

When we think of the good news of the kingdom that Jesus was proclaiming, we need to know that we have all that we need, and it is readily at hand; all we have to do is reach out and get hold of it and use it, because those who are born again have the privilege of living in the kingdom now. I have heard an advocate of healing describe being healed now as 'borrowing' from the kingdom that is to come when Jesus comes back to rule on the earth. That seems to miss the truth that we live in the kingdom now, we are not borrowing it from the future.

It was comforting to find that many eminent scholars and ministers entertained this same understanding about the kingdom and the importance of accepting it as being concurrent with Christian life now. Jean Darnell describes it as 'life in the overlap'; Schweitzer referred to the 'interim ethic'; Gustaf Aulen affirmed that justification was the atonement brought into the present, so that here and now God's blessing would prevail over the curse; J V Taylor suggested that a theology of hope was defective if it meant losing our assurance that the kingdom is already a given. Alan Ecclestone has reminded us that kingdom life is to be taken hold of now; J A T Robinson described the new age with the Holy Spirit as being the 'window' into the meaning of God in Christ. That fascinating image of the Holy Spirit as the window into heaven tied in completely with my understanding of our being the earthly end of the funnel of love. God indeed is in his heaven, way above the problems of man, but stored up alongside is all that Jesus won for us on the cross, all the healing and deliverance from sickness and sin, all the abundant life that he has for us. These benefits are ready to be poured out upon us and into us as we can receive them. When someone who is filled and anointed with the Holy Spirit stands with those who are in need, ready to minister in Jesus' name, we become, as it were, part of the funnel that can direct the flow of love. He is the source; we are the funnel.

During that day in Berlin I also learned more about the need to love and appreciate ourselves as God made us and intended us to be. An attractive young lady, who spoke excellent English, came to me. She said that she had a problem called 'clicky hips'. I am quite ignorant of medical terminology and had never heard that term, but she assured me that it was a well-known medical condition. She said that her hips literally clicked as she walked, and that this was painful and could get worse. I asked the Lord about clicky hips and was led to ask her if she had ever wanted to be a boy and resented being a girl. She then told me the story of how her father had wanted her to be a boy, and so she had done all that she could to please him. She had learned how to run like a boy and to throw like a boy so that she could do all the things that boys and their fathers did. I had to ask her if she was willing to say that she was sorry to God for not accepting who she was, for not accepting that she was a female and being appreciative of all that was feminine about herself. She needed to ask God to forgive her for resenting what he had made her, and for not thanking and praising him in her femininity. She needed to forgive her father for not loving her as she was, the precious gift of a daughter, and forgive him for wanting and encouraging her to be something else. This lovely young lady heard this and cried. She asked the Lord to forgive her and she forgave her own father. She came to a place of accepting and loving herself for who she was. Then, as she walked, she knew she was healed. Her hips no longer clicked. She was a lovely young woman and proud to be so.

One wonderful fact about our God and his love is that he is not limited in time or place. It is his will to heal; it flows from his nature.

The resurrection power to dispense all that Jesus died for is available wherever we might be, through the Holy Spirit, as will be witnessed to throughout this book. I have experienced God allowing me to be a funnel of his love, ministering to many different people, with very different needs, in many different countries and places.

Enfolded in Father's loving arms

At a meeting in the USA, a mother brought her sixteen-year-old son to me. He had been in deep depression since the death of his father. He had become withdrawn and seldom spoke to anyone. All that the Lord directed me to do was hug him. As my arms went around him he clasped me tightly to himself. It seemed to me that the boy was experiencing what he had yearned for, for so long, without knowing how to express it or how to get it: to be comforted in his grief, enfolded in Father God's arms. The time passed: five minutes, ten minutes; my leg got cramp, and you know how you start to get all kinds of itches when you stand totally motionless for any length of time! But I knew that I had to hold that position and could not be the first to release the strength of the embrace. We actually stood there for twenty minutes and probably more before I felt his arms start to loosen their hold on me. Gently he withdrew from me. His eyes were bright, his face was light, his stance and demeanour were tall and confident as he turned and smiled at his mother. She grinned as the tears of joy poured down her face. Her son had returned to her. We had been witnesses to the resurrection power that Paul speaks of, in his letter to the Ephesians, as being ours: *...and his incomparably great power for us who believe. That power is like the working of his mighty strength, which he exerted in Christ when he raised him from the dead and seated him at his right hand in the heavenly realms...* (Ephesians 1:19f.).

Later reports confirmed that the depression was gone and the young man was restored to health and went on from there. In this instance no counselling had been required, no prayers uttered, no apparent deliverance ministry needed. Father had held one of his sons reassuringly in his loving embrace.

This is not the only way in which God manifests healing, and reconciliation into the wholeness of Jesus, in people's lives. We will see many other models of his healing ministry. So let me be quite forthright at the outset and say this: I do not 'believe in healing'! That

15

may seem to be a very strange thing to say, for someone absorbed and involved in Jesus' ministry of healing for nearly thirty years, who is the founder of a Christian healing centre, but it is nonetheless true. I am not being pedantic or playing with words. Let me explain what I mean by this. I believe in Jesus as Lord, and therefore that he has *already* healed. He is the Lord who heals me. This is fundamental to the ministry. Jesus said, *"When a man believes in me, he does not believe in me only, but in the one who sent me"* (John 12:44). Jesus teaches us that the work that God has given us to do is to *believe* in the one whom he sent. (See John 6:29.) That is it; that is our work; that is the sum total. We do not have to *believe in healing*. If we truly *believe in Jesus* and concentrate on that fact alone, then everything else will fall into place. Then we just know deep down inside us, without doubt, that God is God; we just know that we are saved; we just know that we are born again; we just know that we have eternal life, and so on and so on; we know the important truths of who and what we are in him. We do not have to study these matters hard or try to work them out —they are givens when we just believe in Jesus. Concentrate on that. I cannot emphasise it too much. Consider Mark 16:15ff., where Jesus commands the disciples to preach the good news, then says that, "Whoever believes and is baptized will be saved" —and promises that they will place their hands on sick people, and they will get well. It says, 'whoever believes'. Whoever believes what? Whoever believes in Jesus, of course! We do not have to believe in laying hands on the sick —with regard to that, all we have to do is do it. We have to believe in Jesus, and he does the healing part; he does the saving part. I do not have to work myself up into a frenzy of excitement or anticipation. I just have to believe (in him) and then do it.

Because of those words in Mark 16:15ff., I know that I can be involved in changing things for others and myself if I believe in Jesus, but if we start to believe in healing *per se*, we are probably entering into the realms of idolatry. In Numbers 21:4–9 we read of the Israelites in the desert being attacked by venomous snakes. Jesus showed us how to understand this: *"Just as Moses lifted up the snake in the desert, so the Son of Man must be lifted up"* (John 3:14). In telling Moses to make the image of the serpent, it seems as though God was making an exception to the second commandment that forbids making the likeness of any creature on earth, so this had to be something of great importance. The people wanted God to remove the problem completely, taking away the serpents. Similarly, most of us wish that all sickness and sin would be simply eliminated. But God gives relief in his way, not ours. His is a more miraculous way, which is not dependent upon man's answers and remedies but requires us to look to him. It is a way that makes sure we humble ourselves and repent, and look up and see that the cure comes from the hand of God, not man. Jewish thought is that it was not the sight of the serpent that effected the cure, but that it lay in the 'looking up' to God. The passage also teaches us that we should not speak against him or his word. Through Moses the law was given; the word of God was brought to the people. Jesus is the word and the word must be lifted up, as we saw in John 3:14f.

That time in the desert may be likened to our time today in the wilderness or desert of this world. In the desert, fiery serpents attacked them. Who was described as the serpent? The devil, of course, and in Revelation 12:3 he is portrayed as 'a great red dragon'. How fitting —the colour of flames. Paul, in Ephesians 6:16, writes of the 'flaming arrows' that the enemy directs at us, and we think immediately of temptation, sin and sickness. So what was the cure? God prescribed the antidote: lifting up the likeness of the problem, and that seems a very strange thing to do. He did not suggest any of the potions, medicines, remedies, sacrifices or anointings common to the time. No, to simply hold up high, on the pole, the bronze serpent, which was the likeness – not a symbol, but a direct likeness – of the problem. Then they had to look up at it. God's solution to our need of salvation may seem just as strange. His solution for the healing of the whole world, for our redemption, and for releasing us from bondage to the serpent, Satan, may seem strange. His solution was to lift Jesus, God incarnate, high upon the cross. Moses, the law bringer, lifted up the pole with the serpent. The law Moses brought was the Scripture, God's word, which told about Jesus, the Messiah, and how the law would be fulfilled. It was the high priest and the Pharisees, the keepers of the law, the teachers of the word, who had Jesus lifted high on the cross, but they did it in ignorance because they did not understand or believe sufficiently the word that they taught. They did not realise that they were bringing about their own desolation and their damnation. They did not realise they were lifting up the one who would be life and healing to all who believed and looked up to the cross. Jesus was on the cross —and Romans 8:3 tells us what God did: *For what the law was powerless to do in that it was weakened by the sinful nature, God did by sending his own Son in the likeness of sinful man to be a sin offering. And so he condemned sin in sinful man.* The representation of all that was wrong with the world, the likeness of the problem, was on the cross, because there Jesus took upon himself all the sickness, all the sin. Jesus was 'made sin' for us. Moses lifted up the bronze serpent, the likeness of the sickness that beset the people. The Jews lifted up the cross, and on it was the likeness of all the sin and sickness, that was, that is, and which is to come. It was so hideous that it had to be hidden from our eyes by absolute darkness. But the Gospel of John starts by encouraging us: the light shall not be overcome by the darkness. The Jews were healed when they looked up to the likeness on the pole in the desert. We are healed when we look up to the likeness on the cross, and see Jesus. In Numbers 21:9 the Hebrew word used for the pole also signifies a standard, signal, banner or sign. Lifting up Jesus is a signal to all people, a banner waving across the sky. Isaiah says, *In that day the Root of Jesse will stand as a banner for the peoples; the nations will rally to him, and his place of rest will be glorious* (Isaiah 11:10). Jesus, lifted up, triumphs over the serpent, bruising his head. The Israelites looked up and lived. When we look up to Jesus and believe in him, we shall not perish in the desert of this world but have everlasting life. Look up to Jesus, not what he gave us, not for the signs and wonders, but for Jesus himself. The writer to the Hebrews exhorts us: *Let us fix our eyes on Jesus, the author and perfecter of our faith, who for the joy set before him endured the cross, scorning its shame, and sat down at the right hand of the throne of God* (Hebrews 12:2). Isaiah wrote: *Turn to me and be saved, all you ends of the earth; for I am God, and there is no other* (Isaiah 45:22). To the Israelites and to us the message was, and is, the same. But look what happened to the Israelites as time went on. The people started to worship the bronze serpent in itself, rather than looking to God for their healing. It is like so many who look to their church, their denomination, as the most important thing, rather than looking at Jesus. They compromise the word to try to effect unity, when we already have unity, if we stay in the word. Only in the word, only in Jesus, can there be true and everlasting unity. So many, like Simon the magician, look to the wonders as the answer. Faith healers and mediums believe in the healing as the evidence. We have to look to Jesus as the fact, whether or not we see the healing. We must not put healing in the place of Jesus himself. In Matthew 12:38, Jesus rebuked those who asked him for a sign: *Then some of the Pharisees and teachers of the law said to him, "Teacher, we want to see a miraculous sign from you."*

He answered, "A wicked and adulterous generation asks for a miraculous sign! But none will be given it except the sign of the prophet Jonah."

We are not to worship signs or put our faith in them. If we believe in him and worship him only, then the signs and wonders, again, are 'givens', following naturally —spiritually. So many times of revival have faded because, for too many people, the signs and wonders and healings became the most central important factor. Jesus gets sidelined by the phenomena, and when that happens the Holy Spirit and the anointing move on. The Holy Spirit reveals Jesus to us, not just signs and wonders.

Once we have believed, we have to speak out. We need to learn not to be afraid of what other people might say or think about us, whether at home or at work. The institutional church at the moment is so concerned about seeking majority approval from non believers that it is losing the thrust of Jesus' commission to preach the gospel and heal the sick. Our concern should not be whether we are being fair to everybody, nor whether we accommodate everyone's wishes. Salvation comes through the acceptance of Jesus and his word, and we cannot compromise that. *There is a judge for the one who rejects me and does not accept my words; that very word which I spoke will condemn him at the last day.* (John 12:48).

So are we going to believe him, and then get on and do what he tells us to do? That is what being involved with Jesus in his ministry of healing is basically about, believing Jesus and not doubting him. Do that and the anointing, the signs and wonders and the healings will certainly follow. 'Holding in love' is another way of describing what we do as the bottom of the funnel of love. *In this way, love is made complete among us so that we will have confidence on the day of judgment, because in this world we are like him* (1 John 4:17). As his love is perfected in us, he wants us to become his arms of love for others. What follows is what happened for Vera, who came to the Centre.

How do you pray with people who are not able to comprehend? How do you minister to people who, because of their illness, whether mental or physical, are not capable of exercising any faith of their own or taking any conscious part in the praying? Vera was like that. She shuffled into the Centre one Thursday evening, leaning on her silver handled cane with one hand and on Bill, a team member, with the other. Arthritis held her in a vice of pain from the top of her head to the soles of her feet, and had done so for three years or so. Walking was reduced to the slowest pace imaginable, and her dog had got fat through lack of exercise. Vera was a Christian, but the pain and the drugs taken to alleviate the symptoms were so strong that at times she was locked inside her own world.

I was teaching on Acts 12:1–12. It tells how an angel came to Peter in prison, where Herod was holding him until the Feast of the Passover was over, and then Herod, the king, would have him beheaded. Herod had recently had James the brother of John put to death by the sword, and when he saw how much this pleased the Jews he was just waiting to see what he could do for an encore and gain greater adulation from the mob. So when he arrested Peter, everyone knew that there was not a thing that his friends could do about it. What could they do, except pray? As Peter was kept in prison, the whole church in the town was praying fervently for Peter's safety and release. But like so many of us in the church today, although they were praying their socks off in an all night prayer session, it seemed as if they had virtually no expectation that Peter could be saved. Can you imagine it? This crowd of personal friends of the Lord himself were all praying together. I can imagine the scene, firstly praise and worship, standing up, arms upraised, shouting and proclaiming the word, glorifying God, singing praises, reciting and singing the psalms. Then they drop to their knees in repentance, silently meditating on the word, remembering the power in the presence of Jesus. Then they begin retelling all the things that they personally had encountered in their travels with the Lord himself, the miracles, the wonders, the healings, the cross, the graves opening up, the resurrection.... But where was their *belief* that night? That very night, the night before he was due to be executed, an angel appeared in Peter's cell with a flash of light. The angel not only shook Peter to rouse him but actually struck him on the side, saying, *"Quick, get up."* Peter was released from the chains that bound him to the guards, and the angel said, *"Put on your clothes and sandals.... Wrap your cloak around you and follow me."* The angel then led Peter past the other three sets of soldiers stationed, on pain of death, to make sure that he could not get out. After clambering over the soldiers beside him, Peter followed the angel past the first guard and then the second guard. The great door in the front of the prison opened by itself. Peter still did not believe it was happening, still thinking he was seeing a vision. We have witnessed something similar to this phenomenon – the person not believing the miracle is happening– so many times in the ministry of healing: a person's body is set free from the sickness that binds, but the brain or the mind take much longer to catch up, and to process and comprehend what the body has received. Somehow or other, Peter, although physically responding to the instructions of the angel, dressing himself and stepping carefully over the bodies of the sleeping soldiers, was not wholly aware of the reality of what was happening. He walked all the way down the road outside the prison before the full recognition and acceptance of his freedom finally penetrated his consciousness and he realised that this was not a vision or a dream but that he was actually free. He was no longer in bondage. His body had responded to that which his mind could not comprehend. Jesus, through his Spirit, had communicated with Peter's spirit. Our bodies often reflect what is happening in our spirit long before our minds can take it all in. We see people released physically from the bondage of illness and pain before their souls can incorporate it into their consciousness.

Peter decided to go at once to Mary's house. Before she even opens the door, Rhoda the servant girl recognises Peter's voice and, in her excitement, forgets to let him in, dashing back to tell the others he was there! Then comes what for me is one of the craziest pieces of reasoning in the Bible: rather than believe God would answer their prayers, they decide it must be Peter's angel at the door. Eventually, after Peter's insistent knocking continued unabated, they opened the door. I find it quite amazing that these great warriors of prayer, who had learned from the master that nothing is impossible to God, could actually pray so fervently for so long without the practical belief that God would answer them. But it taught me a lot about the efficacy of prayer in obedience to the instructions of Jesus, even when the faith available is tinier than a mustard seed. It shows us clearly that, when we pray and follow his instructions, his grace flows freely and generously in power to anoint the prayer —and the anointing breaks the yoke.

Peter was set free; but what about Vera? To contain the pain and the arthritic symptoms, she had to take prescription drugs which induced sleepiness. So during my talk, and the prayer time which followed, Vera heard not a word for, as far as we were aware, she was in a deep sleep in her chair. When we came to the time for praying with people, I approached Vera and asked whether she could stand. Rather as in Peter's case, her body responded as if in a dream. With assistance, she rose to her feet, standing up very slowly and carefully, as arthritis sufferers and those with acute back pain learn to do, carefully guarding themselves from the pain of sudden movement. When she was on her feet I gently wrapped my arms around her, not speaking or explaining but just holding her in love, in the window of heaven. After some time of holding her, I asked Vera what parts of her body she could move. Slowly she moved her fingers, still holding the cane. I could see her face begin to relax, but it was obvious that her mind was not accepting this. My wife said, "Take her for a walk of faith." Our prayer room is only about eight metres wide, so it was not going to be a long walk. She was encouraged to walk a few steps, very gently at first. I asked Vera to move her head, lift her arms, turn her body, and she responded to all these requests. Then, as she did so, her mind slowly started to grasp the fact that her body was doing all of these things WITHOUT PAIN. Her mouth started to smile and her eyes cleared.

A lady who had been healed at the Centre just two weeks earlier was present on this evening. Her leg had been injured years earlier in an accident. Sadly, the bones had not set correctly, resulting in her right leg below the knee angling out to the right, causing pain and discomfort. At the previous meeting Jesus had straightened this leg and released her from pain. Now she took Vera's hands and said, "Come on, let's run and dance together," and they did so, much to everyone's amusement and joy. Vera was completely set free.

A nurse who had told me at the beginning of the meeting that she was very sceptical about 'healing ministries' was present that night. She worked each day in hospital wards with terminally ill patients. She told me that she had known that Vera's body was riddled right through with arthritis, but even though she had seen her released from the pain of its grip, she still could not really believe it. Would it last?

I referred her to the lady with whom Vera was dancing. At the end of the evening the nurse was standing outside when it came time for Vera to leave. She saw Vera come to the top of the two steps down to the path and watched as Vera paused, turned sideways and then slowly lowered one leg down to the next step, and then the other even more slowly. Vera then repeated this slow and painful looking operation for the second step. You could see the nurse thinking, 'I knew it would not last.' Dorothy asked Vera what she was doing. Vera caught herself and said, "I don't need to do that, do I?" then turned round, ran up the steps and danced down them again. So often, when Jesus heals our bodies, our minds still cling on to old patterns and the behaviour we have learned over years of coping with pain. We need to learn to renew our minds as well. Our bodies have practised and become accustomed to certain habits of behaviour. Both minds and bodies need to be taught again how to move in freedom.

Although Vera had been set free in the prayer room, as Jesus poured his love into her through the Holy Spirit, as through an open window, I wanted to ensure that her healing would remain. I did not want Satan to have any right or reason to be able to steal her health from her again. When we see people lose the ground that they have gained there is usually an underlying reason. So as we drank coffee together before she left, I asked Vera when the arthritis had started. She told me that the arthritis and pain had set in three years earlier, following the death of her wonderful husband, who had meant everything to her; she had worshipped him. This gave me a clue to the problem, and the opening that the illness had been given. God tells us about the sin of idolatry and says that we should have no other gods before him. Worship of any other thing or being is wrong. This can be a difficult subject to broach without arousing anger or disquiet. But Vera's heart wanted to serve the Lord and she understood that it was not good for her to give to her husband and his memory those things which belonged to God. As I led her in prayer, Vera asked God to forgive her for any way in which she had put her husband before him. Then she fully released her husband into God's love and care, as he knew and understood the great love which she had for her husband, and the grief and loss she had felt at his death. We asked the Lord to be her support. Months later, Vera came and gave testimony in our church. We all laughed as she told how her dog was tired out and unhappy because now she walked five miles each day at such a pace that he found it difficult to keep up. He was slim and fit again because whereas in the old days he had waddled alongside Vera as she dragged herself along at a snail's pace, now he had to run. On the first few trips Vera had had to carry him the last part of the way home because he just could not make it.

All that took place several years ago. Recently Vera visited the Centre again. She looked very trim and announced that she was now 74 years of age and had just come from her aerobic classes. Vera's silver handled cane hangs in our prayer room; she never needed it again.

We went to Gateshead

One Sunday morning I preached at a friend's church in Gateshead. After the service he asked me to go and speak to a young lady still sitting in one of the pews. A healthcare professional, she had not been able to work for some time because she was in pain with arthritis and her fingers were stiff so she could not use her hands to massage. I was aware that the arthritis was able to bind because there was unforgiveness and guilt in the situation. As she declared her willingness to forgive, and accepted God's forgiveness, she started to cry, and so did a lady in the pew behind. I later found that the second lady was her mother, who was very concerned for her daughter. As she forgave and sobbed, I could see the release from pain come into her face —but how to get her mind to accept what had happened for the body? Just then a man from the congregation walked past the end of the pew and said, "Good morning."

Involuntarily, the girl turned her head to the side, smiled at him and said, "Cheerio." Then you could clearly see the light dawn in her eyes as she realised what she had done: she had turned her head to the side and it had not hurt. Now she had the courage to try more. I encouraged her to release her hold on the back of the pew in front of her. As she loosened her grip she started to wiggle her fingers; they were free. Then she bent and stretched and enjoyed the feeling. "Oh," she said, as her mother and I began to laugh, "I will be able to go home and peel the potatoes for the Sunday dinner!"

2

SPEAKING TO FAITH

In the last chapter I broached the subject of faith and the difficulties and fears that this can arouse in the minds and hearts of ministers and churchgoers in relation to Christian healing. Will they have enough faith? Have they got enough faith? Will they be found wanting? How about non-churchgoers and non-Christians? Do they have faith or need to have faith to be healed? Let us look at this more closely. We start with the story of a coal miner.

He came to Beggars Roost

Towards the end of one August in the early 1990s, some of his friends brought a man we will call Matthew to one of our weekly Thursday evening services of prayer for healing. Matthew, who was in his early forties, did not have a relationship with Jesus, nor did he come with any expectancy that he might be healed. It came to the time in the service when we offer ministry. His friends prompted him to come forward. Matthew told me that his occupation from his youth had been as a miner at the coalface. This was a tough, physical, dirty job. The mines in Northumberland and Durham were deep with very low, narrow, damp seams. Once a miner left the lift shaft cage that took him underground he had to stoop, creep or crawl over the cold, wet, black surface for the duration of his shift. When Matthew was 23 he was diagnosed as having 'ankylosis spondylitis'. The first term has been defined as 'abnormal adhesion or immobility of the bones in a joint as by direct joining of the bones'; the latter as 'inflammation of the vertebrae'. This must have been devastating news for Matthew and the implications for his life were horrendous. It meant that, starting from the bottom, the bones in his spine had already started to fuse together. At the prime of his manhood, Matthew knew that as the years went by the disease would travel upwards, fusing one vertebra after another to the one above. His backbone would become increasingly rigid, making it impossible for him to bend or flex his back. After 15 years even his strong determination to work could not beat the disease. When he could no longer bend to move through the low coal seams he had to leave work. One can imagine the torment that had lived within his mind and body over those years, knowing that inevitably his spine would be like a an iron rod, petrified into permanent inflexibility. Doctors and medical specialists consider this to be irreversible, incurable. This is how Matthew was brought to the Centre, with no hope, no future, no job, no life worth living.

We stood facing each other in the centre of the prayer room floor as he told me his story. I sought Father God in prayer. Matthew needed to know how Jesus loved him so much that he lived and died that he, Matthew, might have eternal life; that Father God knew him and wanted him, and that to him Matthew had always been and always would be unconditionally acceptable; that God had heard the hurt and anguish in his spirit through the years; that on the cross Jesus took into himself the sin and sickness of the whole world. It was a delight to lead Matthew in a prayer asking Jesus into his life. I then ministered to Matthew three times as the Holy Spirit prompted me. The first things to be dealt with were the fears that had beset him over the years. Then there was the dread in his mind of not being able to work and provide for his family. Twice, as I spoke into the fears and the dreads within him, the Holy Spirit overwhelmed him and gently laid him out on the carpet. I presume that as he lay supine the Holy Spirit ministered the love of Jesus directly to his spirit. He went down a third time as I spoke to the physical condition. On this occasion when he fell to the floor I knelt with him and held the back of his head in the palm of my hand. His spine had set in such a way that his head was permanently angled forward, with the result that when he lay on his back his head was always six inches from the floor. No exertion on his part could bring his head into contact with the floor. He told me afterwards that in bed he had always had to use a high pillow to get any comfort. As I held his head it gradually sank lower and lower as the Lord un-fused the spine. After about ten minutes I could feel the back of my hand touching the carpet. I gently withdrew my hand until the back of his head was resting on the carpet. It took a while for this to register in Matthew's consciousness, and then he quietly said, "It's touching; my head is touching the floor." He lay a long time, seemingly letting his mind and body assimilate this marvellous thing which had just happened. When he eventually got to his feet I asked him to sit down on a chair with his legs stretched forward. As I held his ankles, the Lord released his hips. When he next stood up he could turn his neck, wiggle his hips and bend down. Others in the team then ministered with him for strengthening of his muscles and so on. He was a different man when he left —and he was born again.

I am not a 'healer'

People who come to the Northumbrian Centre of Prayer for Christian Healing, or others who hear me speak at meetings elsewhere, often ask: 'Are you a faith healer?' My answer always has to be no. I am not a 'healer'. Jesus is the healer, and I simply minister his love. But the questions are raised: 'Do you have to believe to get healed?', and, 'Do you have to consciously have faith?' Matthew, when he came to us, had no belief or expectancy for his healing. We must remember that faith and belief can signify very different things, even though we might hear so many sermons which treat them as synonymous. The problem with most of us is not whether we have faith but how we invest it. Everyone of us has faith, but just think of what we normally do with it. Think of the things that we say, such as: 'If I organise a barbecue for Saturday it will probably rain'; or, 'I can't believe like that'; or, 'Winter is coming on, I will probably get a cold. I usually catch whatever is going around' —and so on and so on.

Often we get what we expect, even if we find it hard to invest in biblical expectation. But we have 'a measure of faith'. (See Romans 12:3). Therefore when I preach or teach on healing or when I pray with people for healing, although I speak in words and sentences that people can understand intellectually, I am not primarily speaking to their minds. Their minds often cannot take it in, or because of their experience their minds cannot accept it. I am speaking into their faith. This is why it is a good thing, when praying for someone, to pray aloud: we are not telling God what to do, but are speaking into faith.

This is why it is not daft, whether interceding for someone thousands of miles away, or in the house round the corner, to speak out our prayers for them aloud, even though there is not the remotest chance that they might hear what we are praying. In creation God spoke the word, and worked through the power of the Spirit who moved over the face of the waters. Jesus was the word made flesh. One key biblical definition of faith is this: *Now faith is being sure of what we hope for and certain of what we do not see* (Hebrews 11:1). The word used for hope is *elpizo*, meaning 'to expect with desire'. Therefore I speak into faith expectantly, not with a forlorn hope but with an expectant desire to see people healed. I then watch in awe, not in surprise, to see what Jesus has done. This is not the proof of my faith, but it proves that what God says about faith is true.

Jesus has already healed by his stripes and death on the cross. When we speak into faith and see the lame walk or ankylosis spondylitis healed, that which already was fact is now seen to be the case. Speaking into faith is one aspect of 'absorption theology' which I have termed my understanding of healing theology, to distinguish it from other theologies. On the cross Jesus took all sickness and disease from past, present and future onto himself. He already has won our healing. But how do we appropriate it?

We went to Beverley, Yorkshire

One evening I was the guest speaker at a dinner being held by the Full Gospel Businessmen's Fellowship International in Beverley, Yorkshire. During my talk I mentioned Matthew's healing. Immediately the time for ministry started, a man came forward who had suffered for years from the same problem. Again as I spoke to the condition his spine started to 'unfreeze'. For some reason that night the healing was only about 98%; his head was still a whisper from the floor. After I had been ministering to others, his wife came up to me in tears. But these were tears of happiness. For the first time for years her husband had been able to take her in his arms and not only cuddle her tight but look into her eyes at the same time.

We went to Hanbury Manor[1]

The time when we went to Hanbury Manor is a good example of the time or place being of no consequence in relation to receiving healing from Jesus. Although the people we were with had no faith as far as

28

they knew, and in the main were not churchgoers, we witnessed what was called *Signs and Wonders on the Tenth Tee* when featured in the May 1996 edition of *Renewal*. Let me start some time before the actual weekend. I was ordained into the priesthood with the intention that I would represent the church in the workplace. Perhaps my understanding of taking the anointing into the world of commerce was slightly different from that of many of my colleagues. I understand Luke 5:17 to be telling us that where Jesus is, then the power to heal is present, and this is irrespective of situation. We should be walking at all times in the anointing. Quite a number of years ago, my son David and I went to the sumptuous Hanbury Manor for a weekend to attend the AGM of the 'Hairdressing Manufacturers and Wholesalers Association' (HMWA). In our secular business, which is a family firm called Rand Rocket Ltd., we are major suppliers of hairdressing scissors to the professional trade. Both David and I were Council members of the Association, so it was our duty to attend such meetings. Signs and wonders of healings are usually associated in most people's minds with special church services, big rallies or villages in central Africa where they cannot afford the doctors' fees for medical treatment. But we must always thank God for his impartiality and his desire to be with us when invited. On this extremely hot afternoon in May, as a young man landed his helicopter on the lawn to pick up his sister who was playing tennis with her girl friend, the Lord manifested his first amazing healing —on the tenth tee of the verdant golf course. At these annual events, after the first part of the business meeting on the Saturday morning, David and I try to find time to mix with the other delegates, many of whom are customers, and if possible we play golf with them.

It was on the first tee that I remarked on the very short back swing of Martin Woodgate, one of the fourball match that we were playing. This, he told us, was due to the fact that he had injured his right shoulder some four years ago. Despite visits to doctors and physiotherapists over the years, his shoulder had been written off as incurable. So he had geared his life and his golf to working within the limited movement this allowed him. It was on the tenth tee that I was finally prompted to say, "Martin, your shoulder can be healed." Once again he patiently explained about the doctors and the physiotherapists, and the impossibility of this. "Not the doctors, but Jesus can heal that today," I replied.

29

Without blinking an eyelid, he replied, "Go on then."

First I asked him to stretch out his arms straight in front of him, as I usually do with such problems, and then told his arms and his back and all the muscles and joints to come into alignment and be made whole. By this time David had taken the opportunity to slip quietly behind Martin, and stood in readiness for the next part. As I reached out to hold Martin's neck to deal with that, I told him not to worry if he fell over. "Why..." came from his lips as he fell, wide-eyed, backwards, under the anointing of the Holy Spirit, into David's arms, and was gently lowered to the grass, where he lay for five minutes or more. The fourth member of our group just stood open-mouthed and speechless as he witnessed Jesus at work, then he turned away, seeming to pretend that nothing untoward had happened and really he was not with us. Martin lay motionless. I kept watch to see if the next fourball was catching up, but God was with us because, although the course was busy, we were completely undisturbed. Then, somewhat shaky and bewildered, Martin climbed to his feet and began testing his arm and shoulder: first his arm high above his head, then round and up behind his back, into a position I have never been capable of achieving even when young. "I haven't been able to do that for five years," he murmured, an incredulous grin of delight on his face.

"I have never been able to do that," I replied. Martin was flabbergasted. Full mobility had been restored, there was no pain, and he executed the most demanding manoeuvres with his arms. As Martin was partnering my son David against a friend and myself, I was delighted to see that his game went completely to pot as he tried to work out a new swing! Over the next eight holes it did not take a particularly keen observer to notice how he constantly raised his arm in the air and stuck his hand up behind his back. Where the first nine holes had been fairly even, my partner and I were clear victors on the back nine. But this was not to be the end of the witness to Jesus on this beautiful spring weekend. Martin was just too full of his wonderment at what had happened to him to keep it a secret. As I bought drinks at the bar, he was out on the balcony above the pro-shop, regaling everyone there with an account of the proceedings on the tenth tee, showing them in detail the wonderful things that he could now do with his right arm that he had not been able to do for five years.

"What about my knees, then?" a pretty young lady, with long

legs, which were elegantly revealed by the shorts she was wearing, said to me as I emerged from the bar. She explained that she had problems with both knees and that nothing could be done for them. This time, as she fell under the anointing of the Holy Spirit, onto the stone floor of the veranda, there was a large crowd of witnesses wanting an explanation of what was happening. This gave us more opportunities to tell about Jesus.

The dinner dance held that evening was preceded by a reception. When we entered the hall where the reception was being held I immediately spotted Martin. He was sharing his good news with more members of the Association, demonstrating with grand gestures all the movement that had been restored to him that afternoon on the golf course. Jim Dallas, President of the Association, came over to me. He mentioned that he had suffered from headaches for forty years, and asked whether prayer would help him. Jim is a very tall, well-built man. My son David, who is five feet seven inches, when he saw from the bar what was going on, moved into position behind Jim. David was busy praying that Jim would not fall under the Spirit. Although the Holy Spirit came powerfully on Jim and he swayed back and forwards, to David's relief (and probably his own) he did not go down. He did remark, however, on the tingling sensation, and the peace and relief that he felt.

At this, Richard, the Secretary of the Association, came up beside me and informed me of how he had suffered with arthritis in his knees and feet for many, many years. Even the bones in his feet were now disfigured. At this point I spied a door leading off the reception room. When I opened it, I found an office that was temporarily vacant. The Lord gave me a word of knowledge about the origin of Richard's arthritis. Again, after praying about this, he fell to the floor under the power of the Holy Spirit and lay there for a considerable time. I kept praying that the owner of the office would not return before we were ready, because it would take quite a bit of explaining as to why I had a motionless body at my feet. Eventually Richard 'came to', and I helped him to his feet. He flexed his knees and tried out things which would normally have caused him pain and announced that the pain had all gone, and we thanked Jesus for it. David told me the following day that when talking with Richard, late into the night, he was still professing what had happened for him, and showing how the bones in his feet had now returned to their proper shape.

Fairly soon after Richard and I left the office the announcement was made that we should proceed to the dining room. As I took my place at the dining table, a lady moved to a seat beside me. Richard actually worked for her husband's company. She said that Richard had told her of the wonderful thing that had happened for him. She asked if it would be possible for me to pray with her, as the arthritis in her legs had grown worse and worse, particularly over the past two years, to the point where her mobility was greatly impaired. Anne was a churchgoing Christian in her sixties. She and her husband loved to travel, but the joys of travel and life in general were being more and more restricted by this encroaching disablement. We agreed that after the dinner we would get together and bring the problem before the Lord. The meal was delightful and the company and conversation were excellent, so it was not until well after midnight that I was able to gather Anne and her husband, together with Martin and his wife Carole. Martin had told us how his wife suffered with pain in her lower back and hips and he was eager for her to experience the release and relief that he had. So Anne waited with eager anticipation as Carole explained that nothing could be done about her problem with her lower back and hips, and that this was something that she simply had to live with and that really she had learned to cope very well. I explained that to God nothing was impossible and all she could lose was her pain, and suggested that we proceeded on that basis. First, with her arms stretched out in front, I commanded her back and arms to come into alignment —which they did. Attention was then transferred to her lower back and pelvic region, which were ordered to come back into place, with the muscles and tissues strengthened and repaired. I told the pain to leave her. Then, as I ministered to her neck and vertebrae, asking the Holy Spirit to come as the oil of anointing right down her spine, she fell under the power of the Spirit. On climbing to her feet after resting and soaking in the Spirit for some time, I asked her to show me what she had not been able to do. As she bent down and twisted her hips vigorously, we thanked Jesus.

Anne tentatively stood for prayer, and I realised that she needed a 'full alignment'. First, as with Carole, I got her to stretch her arms out straight in front, and commanded the whole of the back area to come into alignment. As I then lightly touched her neck to open up all the arteries and veins and communication of the brain with the rest of the body, she fell under the Spirit for the first time. After a while I asked her to sit straight in an upright chair and hold out her legs in front of her. This was still a painful exercise for Anne at this stage. As I supported her ankles it was clearly visible to all in the room that the left heel and ankle were about one and a half inches higher than on the right leg. With everybody observing, so that they would not miss the marvellous thing that Jesus was going to do, I commanded the hips and the legs to come into the proper alignment in Jesus' name. For once the reaction was virtually instantaneous. The left leg moved smoothly into alignment so that the heels and the anklebones corresponded exactly with those of the right leg. Then, as she stood, I spoke to the lower back and pelvic area and she went down again under the Spirit. I asked the Lord to fill her with peace and joy. Eventually, when she was able to stand, I asked her to do the things that had been difficult before, and she was able to do these without pain. "What was the most difficult of all?" I asked. She told how stairs had been the biggest bugbear, and how she had had to tackle them sideways on, always getting both feet onto each stair before proceeding to the next. So I suggested that we go and find some stairs to try out her new mobility.

One o'clock in the morning saw five of us marching down the hotel corridor to the nearest staircase, which turned out to be also the steepest. Bravely, Anne approached the stairs directly, face on. She lifted her foot to the first stair and then immediately her other foot to the second stair, and so on, straight up the staircase. Up she went, one foot after the other, one stair after the other, without pause. At the top she turned round with a triumphant smile on her face. I asked her what the second most difficult thing was. "Going down stairs", she replied. She needed no encouragement to start on this second most difficult thing to do. Anne descended the staircase facing forwards without holding the banister. No turning sideways and gently lowering each foot from step to step: at the bottom she was triumphant; she turned round and did it all over again, up and down. Their bedroom was upstairs, so she had to climb a third time as everyone said goodnight. Next morning I followed some fifty yards behind Anne as they walked from the Garden Court, where our bedrooms were, through the grounds to the main hotel, where breakfast was served. It was good to see her walking straight, the rolling gait gone, and then down the stone steps without hesitation.

The six people directly touched by the Lord on that spring Saturday were aware of the reality of the physical presence of Jesus and were undoubtedly affected. Many others saw and witnessed his signs and wonders. At breakfast, Martin and Carole discussed where they could go to church in York.

Jesus can meet people and heal them in the workplace

The only proviso is that we have to be brave and speak up, knowing that we are living in the kingdom. Again we are talking about people with no thought of having faith. For instance, one day in my office, in an old building that we rented in Hitchin, I was negotiating advertising space with the representative (whom I will call Peter) of a trade magazine. As he moved to pick up his folder I saw him wince with pain. He explained that he had problems with his back. I told him that Jesus could heal that if he wanted him to. Peter nodded politely and carried on with his sales spiel. When the contracts were signed and he was ready to go, I again gave him the opportunity to get rid of the pain. This time, probably as I was the customer and it is usually a good sales ploy to humour your customers, he agreed. Much to his surprise, I simply told the pain to go in the name of Jesus and it went. He stretched and stretched and he went home smiling, pain free. A few days later I received a note confirming the contract and asking me to thank 'the boss' for his back.

About a year later I was walking through the main concourse of the National Exhibition Centre (NEC). This is a massive series of commercial exhibition halls near Birmingham, and every year the International Spring Fair occupies every inch of available space. My company had exhibited at this exhibition every year since the NEC was built. The main concourse was crowded, but I spotted Peter walking towards me. He stopped and said that he had been to our stand to find me for two reasons. One was to negotiate next year's advertising contract and the other was to ask for prayer for his back. It had all been great until the previous week when he had strained it. The pain had returned and he would like prayer again. "However," he said, looking at the jostling crowd around us, "there is probably a time and place for everything." I promised him that wherever we were was the right time and place, so we then moved to the side of the concourse and I prayed for his back to be healed. Again the release was instantaneous and he thanked Jesus and me. Shyly, he told me that his two daughters went to guides at the local Methodist church but that he only went on special occasions and supposed he ought to go more often. I took the opportunity to invite Peter and his wife to one of the dinners that the Full Gospel Businessmen's Fellowship International (FGBMFI) held every month in Hitchin. Possibly because he was so grateful for the release from pain, he agreed to come. As it turned out I was unable to get to the dinner that month, so Dorothy stood in as host for all our guests that evening. Peter asked Jesus to be Lord in his life at the dinner. I received a note of thanks from him. A few days after receiving it, Dorothy answered a phone call from his wife. Peter had had a heart attack and died suddenly. He had come home from work and was playing table tennis with his daughters when he fell over the table, and was dead. Dorothy found herself dumbfounded and stupidly asking whether she was sure he was dead. Peter was dead all right, and his wife had phoned to thank us for all we had done. She was a Christian and she knew that Peter had been born again at the dinner and so he, too, was Christian. Now she and the girls had the joy of knowing that he was now in heaven with Jesus, and that one day they would see Peter again. Therefore they could cope with the loss and the grief, as a family, in a much more confident way than would have been possible just the week before. She also knew that some of the money that Peter had left them had to be used to invite other men to dinners and help lead them to Jesus.

We should never be embarrassed to talk about Jesus because of the place we are in, or the people we are with. It is by the witness of his power to heal that so many can come to recognise the reality of his presence in this world and their need for him.

We went to Solingen, Germany

One day I had taken my sales force to Germany to visit the factory in Solingen, to see how our hairdressing scissors were manufactured and to keep them up to date with some of the new technologies that we were using to keep us ahead of our competitors. As we walked through the factory I noticed that one of our sales managers who was walking in front of me seemed to be a bit 'lopsided' as he walked. I called to him and got him to stop while I asked him about this. It turned out that he had always had a slight limp. Right there, in the middle of the workshop with all the men looking on, I got him to sit down on one of the workbenches. With his permission I took hold of his ankles and raised his feet off the ground. I placed the thumb of each hand on the centre of each anklebone. It was immediately apparent that they were out of alignment by about an inch. This did not necessarily mean that one leg was longer than the other; through personal experience with my own hips, I know that one hip can sort of get caught up on the hip joint. The practitioner who has unhooked my own left hip on at least a couple of occasions told me this. He had a more medical sounding explanation, but that is what it seemed to me that he was describing. The sales manager could see the difference clearly, and he watched as I commanded his legs to come into alignment in the name of Jesus. And they did. He was quite amazed at what he had seen and felt, and when he stood up and we carried on with the factory tour he no longer had a lopsided gait.

A lady was released from spondylosis, to leap and dance and praise the Lord. She came to a Thursday evening service with friends. She was ministered to by Margot and David, two of our team, and was completely healed from that condition. When they ministered to her, the Holy Spirit put her flat out on the floor, where she lay for a long time. She subsequently wrote and told me that she knew she was healed the moment she was able to rise from the floor unaided. I was involved elsewhere, and looked round to see who the woman was who was shouting, singing and dancing. She was doing all the things that she could not do: touching her toes bending from the hips; raising her knees high as she danced; and, above all, stretching up her arms to wave her hands in the air as she praised the Lord. She and her friends did not stop dancing, singing and praising for about an hour or more, and would not have stopped then if we had not needed to close for the night. Afterwards she described to me the condition that she was in when she arrived that Thursday. She told me that it was as if she had a steel bar right across her shoulders, another down her spine, and another across her hips. She was in great pain all the time and could not bend her arms, lift her arms above a certain height, or look over her shoulders. Her hips were stiff and sore and walking was very difficult. She could not lie flat on the floor and certainly would not have been able to get up again. She could not go anywhere alone as she would only be able to shuffle after a short distance. She would get dizzy and had pins and needles in both her arms and legs. She could black out if she looked upwards. In her letter to me she said that since getting home she has been going out into Newcastle alone and unaided, and that she suffered no more from the pain that had been her constant companion.

Upside down prayer

I was thinking about prayer and faith and I got this silly picture in my mind of 'upside down' prayer —of how so many of us seem to stand on our heads to pray! We pray from the problem rather than pray from the solution. We pray with our heads deep in the problem or deep in the mire, instead of from the throne room.

To him who overcomes, I will give the right to sit with me on my throne, just as I overcame and sat down with my Father on his throne (Revelation 3:21). *And God raised us up with Christ and seated us with him in the heavenly realms in Christ Jesus* (Ephesians 2:6). *Who is it that overcomes the world? Only he who believes that Jesus is the Son of God* (1 John 5:5). That is us! If you believe in Jesus as Lord, then you are an overcomer. I think that my favourite book in the Bible is Ephesians. If you read it you see that it is written in retrospect, from the point where everything is already done. *Praise be to the God and Father of our Lord Jesus Christ, who has blessed us in the heavenly realms with every spiritual blessing in Christ* (Ephesians 1:3). He **has** blessed us. Not will bless us – or might bless us – or will possibly or probably bless us. He has blessed us; it is a given, an already done deal. Paul goes on to pray that the eyes of our hearts may be 'enlightened' so that we may know the hope to which God has called us. (See 1:18.) How does God do this? *For it is by grace you have been saved, through faith—and this not from yourselves, it is the gift of God...* (Ephesians 2:8).

If this is a gift, and it is something that we did not do for ourselves, do we just sit back now and let God get on with all the rest? Not at all. Jesus is the head; we are the body. The function of the body is to do what the head tells it to do. We keep on asking Jesus to do things for us when we should be doing them ourselves. One reason we do not, is because so many of us do not think that we have the power to do anything that is of real importance or significance. However, I ask you to consider this verse: *Now to him who is able to do immeasurably more than all we ask or imagine, according to his power that is at work within us...* (Ephesians 3:20). Note that it refers to his power that is at work within us. Jesus has already dealt with the problem of our feeling weak and helpless. He has put his power to work and he has put it to work inside us. Therefore we need to learn how to use that power.

The next objection and problem many of us raise concerns faith. 'Oh,' we say, 'this takes faith; I need faith.' If we are saved, how did we get saved? Scripture tells us that we are saved by grace, through faith. If you are saved, then you must have faith. Salvation is a gift; grace and faith go together, for we see when we have received Christ that the saving faith we were given in fact came by grace.

Somehow many feel, quite mistakenly, that faith is the power to make God do things, and that if we had enough we could get God to do anything. But faith does not make God do anything. Faith is a positive response to what God has already done by grace. I hear so much wrong teaching of the 'name it and claim it' variety, which suggests that if we just keep on confessing something out, if we keep on claiming something, or thinking 'now I am standing in faith, this will eventually move God to do something about it', that this will surely make him respond. Or we feel that if we say it hard enough and often enough, he will eventually intervene and do something: he will intervene and I will be healed. This seems to me to come into the category of prayer that we are warned about in Matthew 6:7, *"And when you pray, do not keep on babbling like pagans, for they think they will be heard because of their many words."* Because of this type of teaching, I meet so many disillusioned Christians. I meet ministers and members of congregations who are adamantly opposed to anything to do with the healing ministry because, in their experience, it does not work. They have claimed healing for themselves, or for a loved one, for what seemed like an eternity, and to them God seemed to be ignoring them. They do not understand the authority which God has given to those who believe. I look at the issue of authority in greater depth later. Simply claiming something does not make it faith, and even if it were, faith can only appropriate what God has already done by grace.

Whilst it is certainly true that we must confess the truth of the word, we first have to find out what God has already provided with regard to the particular situation, problem or circumstance we are bringing to him. However, in the case of healing we know that he has already provided healing. Most of us are trying to command or persuade God to do something he has already done. It is not that God *can* heal but that he already *has* healed. If we buy or make something and we have it in our possession, we do not doubt that we have it, we *know* we have it. We need to come into this same place of knowing with regard to healing. The doubts come in with healing because we are still battling to get it —when we already have it, but cannot see it! Sometimes when the manifestation of the healing does not happen in a specific time period, the tendency is to wonder whether we ever are going to receive it. Think of electric power. The power is continuously pouring through the cables from the generators to our homes. To light the lamp we have to turn on the switch or plug in the connector. If the lamp does not light, we do not immediately think that the power station has stopped generating power. We accept that the fault is at our end and change the bulb or the fuse. But so often we think that God has stopped reaching out to us or talking to us, when really it is we who have stopped listening to him.

We are reminded that *we who have believed* have entered the 'rest' which is of God. (See Hebrews 4:3.) This is a 'given', but is not entered into if hearing is not combined with faith. No-one can 'go into' it if they are living in disobedience. So you need to speak the word, the truth of what he did on the cross, into the faith that is within you. Let the word enter in; believe, walk in obedience to Jesus, trust his words and rest in him. As the word enters in, we move closer into Jesus and all that he has already done. God's promises in his word assure us that, if we do what he has asked us to do, he will provide. As we enter into his rest, we can pray, 'Lord you have already healed me; now what do you want me to do?'

Sandra came to Beggars Roost

She wrote: *In 1997, on my first visit to the Healing Centre, Randy announced that the Lord was going to heal someone of an itching scalp. That happened to be me, and it used to drive me to distraction. Also, on the same visit, I had been involved in a car accident, which damaged my back, I had musculo–ligamentous strain of the lower back. I had prayer, and God healed it too —100%.*

On another visit, in July 1997, my mobility was limited due to a knee injury. The Lord healed my leg so that my mobility was far better than it had been for many years. The following day, when I went to work, my manager told me, out of the blue, that I was to visit every shop in Newcastle over the next few days. (Boy, was I relieved that I felt better that morning). I was sent out first thing and returned to the office at 4.30 p.m. If this event had happened prior to this healing, I would not have made it past lunchtime and would have had to lie down for the rest of the day, as my back and leg would have been very painful and I would have been completely exhausted. After the weekend I was sent out again for another couple of days —Praise God, I was fine!

Note
[1] Part of the Hanbury Manor story was first published in *Renewal*, Issue 240, May 1996 edition.
Now refer to: www.christianitymagazine.co.uk

3

WHAT FAITH DOES A DEAD MAN HAVE?

Many people do not feel that they can expect to be healed, largely because they do not feel that they have enough faith or the right kind of faith. But the teaching of Jesus does not encourage us to depend on what we see and feel, but rather upon the word of God. Like Martha or Mary (in John 11:21,32) we might think that it would be different if only Jesus were actually here. Surely, if he were to be standing right here with us, then we would have faith, then we would ask for healing, and then we would see healing. Then we could be sure. Yet Jesus is of the here and now. Though we do not see him with our physical eyes, he is present because he rose from the dead and is alive now.

In this chapter I want to encourage all who think they do not have enough faith to be healed to move into a new place so that they can receive healing. We will consider that incident in John 11, which describes Lazarus being raised from the dead. Recall the depression that swamped those who loved Lazarus. The chapter opens with the news that Lazarus is sick. His sisters, Martha and Mary, are sending news of this to Jesus who, with his disciples, is staying some distance away from their home at Bethany. Jesus tells the disciples that Lazarus is sick but adds that the sickness will not end in death, and some discussion follows of the meaning of the word 'asleep' which reveals a degree of perplexity on the part of the disciples. What Jesus was about to do would reveal something of the glory and power of God, showing clearly just who Jesus is. What would make you sit up and take notice most: to see someone get better, or to see a dead person get up and walk and talk? The disciples had seen a good deal of healing, but it was necessary that they should move quickly into a deeper understanding of faith and belief. When Jesus told them that they were going to Lazarus, the thoughts of the disciples seem mainly to have centred on themselves. Why? Because last time they were in that area the Jews had tried to stone Jesus. Jesus first told the disciples that Lazarus had 'fallen asleep', using a euphemism for death we still use today, which is used elsewhere in the Bible, and would not have been unknown to the disciples. I find it hard to understand at times why Jesus bothered to hang around with this thick bunch —but then I start to wonder why he bothers with me! He used the word 'asleep' in much the same way when, in Luke 8, we read how he raised Jairus' daughter from death. In any event, Jesus then has to spell it out for them, and clearly state that Lazarus is dead. Then Thomas, a good example of a despondent depressive, maybe thinking of the local people with stones at the ready, says, "Let us also go, that we may die with him." That is the crowd that Jesus is moving with. The only faith and expectation that they have is that they are also going to finish up dead. Jesus finally arrived near Bethany, four days after Lazarus had died. I feel that he waited four days because he wanted all the glory to go to God and to stop any superstitious nonsense from taking any of the glory away. It seems that there was a contemporary idea that a person's spirit hung around for three days after they had died. Therefore it would not have been such a big thing for Lazarus to come to life again within that period, but now after four days Lazarus could be counted as well and truly dead and buried. At Bethany, Jesus finds unbelief and depression, as well as 'if only's. Martha said to Jesus, *"If you had been here, my brother would not have died"* (v. 21).

Attitudes to healing today are often quite similar to those displayed by Thomas and some of those others around Jesus who frequently showed a lack of faith and expectancy. Even Christians with an assurance of salvation sometimes find it hard to believe God's word for now —and it is believing his word for *now* that is the distinctive characteristic of those Christians I want to work with in Jesus' ministry of healing. Millions of Christians filling the church pews believe in Jesus. But even the demons believe in Jesus, inasmuch as they recognize his existence and his power. The big question for me is not whether you 'believe in Jesus' but do you *believe Jesus*? Do you believe what he says? Do you believe he gave authority and power to those he sent out to 'cure diseases'. (See Luke 9:1 and 10:9.) Do you believe Jesus who said, *"Go back and report to John what you hear and see: The blind receive sight, the lame walk, those who have leprosy are cured, the deaf hear, the dead are raised, and the good news is preached to the poor"* (Matthew 11:4ff). Do you agree with Jesus' description of the signs that accompany the life of a Christian? —*"Whoever believes and is baptized will be saved, but whoever does not believe will be condemned. And these signs will accompany those who believe: In my name they will drive out demons; they will speak in new tongues; they will pick up snakes with their hands; and when they drink deadly poison, it will not hurt them at all; they will place their hands on sick people, and they will get well"* (Mark 16:16ff). This is all that I initially ask of those who want to join us in the work of the Northumbrian Centre of Prayer for Christian Healing. I once heard an elderly Pentecostal lady from Jamaica preaching on that passage, and she quoted it as "Whosoever believes and has been baptized...." From then on I could not help but think of myself as a 'whosoever'! Are you a 'whosoever'? Do you believe Jesus? I have never seen the dead raised, but I believe he can do it, and I am waiting for the day that I do see it happen.... If Jesus had taken a vote amongst those who had gathered there, including the disciples, as to how many believed that he could raise Lazarus from the dead, I doubt that even one hand would have been raised. Can you imagine that noisy scene in Bethany as friends gathered around to console the sisters, wailing and weeping with them? And when they saw them move to the tomb, the crowd would have followed them there, expecting more weeping. There may have been hired professional mourners to augment the grief of the relatives and friends. We can imagine how, when they saw Jesus start to cry, those present would have joined in even more loudly. (See v. 33.) They thought that Jesus was crying because his friend Lazarus was dead. But it says that Jesus was troubled in spirit. Can you wonder? It was much the same as when he was weeping over the temple in Jerusalem, the house of God. These were his followers, this was to be his body on earth, and not even they believed him. I think he wept at their lack of faith.

Now we come to the grave and the stone. I think of that stone as representing unbelief, hurts, fears, hatred, anger, rejection and pain. The stone represents a stumbling block. Before we can start moving in faith – from just believing *in* him, which is the start, to doing even greater works than he did – there are stones of varying sizes in all of us which need to be moved. In Matthew 17:20 the stone becomes a mountain, and even then Jesus says that we only need a mustard seed of faith to remove it. Jesus gave instruction to move the stone at the tomb; Mary argued with that. Think of the stench. The body had been there for four days. Can you think of all the problems, all the hurts, all the despair, all the anger, all the fears, all the doubts, the rejection, the domination, the hatred, that you have not been able to deal with over the years, that you have just pushed, deeper and deeper, down inside yourself until you think it has been hidden and buried, but it just lies festering and messing up your life today? That is the sort of stench that I mean. These are the stones that we are too frightened even to look at, never mind move. But Jesus wants us to be healed; Jesus wants the real us – the real you, the real me –brought to life. So *we* have to remove the stones. Recall how Jesus said to Martha that if she believed she would see the glory of God (John 11:40); if we want to see the glory of God then 'removing the stone' is indeed the only way. *We* have to do that removing. Now Martha starts to move beyond her own reasoning. She moves past thinking; she moves past doubting. To move into faith we have to move past what our minds, which have been trained to be sceptical, can even envisage. This is why Paul in Ephesians 1:18 prays that the eyes of the readers' *hearts* will be enlightened. The stone is removed. At that point Martha had moved into the next stage of obedience and doing what Jesus said, for no other reason than that he said it. If you get that far, then you are ready to start to come into Jesus' ministry of healing.

Then Jesus prayed to the Father. *So they took away the stone. Then Jesus looked up and said, "Father, I thank you that you have heard me. I knew that you always hear me, but I said this for the benefit of the people standing here, that they may believe that you sent me"* (John 11:41f).

Jesus knew that not only was he heard then, but that he was always heard. He had that great assurance of unconditional acceptance by the Father that he wants us to have. Do you know that the Father has always heard you and that he still hears you every time you speak to him? But we still need to remove those stones, and then there is so much more he can do for us. After prayer, Jesus spoke to the problem. He said, *"Lazarus come out!"* He gave this comand in a loud voice. That was so appropriate. By contrast, I think of some prayer groups where everybody mutters their prayers just below the threshold for hearing, and then expects others to say 'Amen.' How can I? I do not know whether I agree. Incidentally, I implore you never to say 'Amen' to anything you have either not heard or do not agree with. Nor should you assent to any vague, 'whatever is your will' type of prayer, because prayer is to ask Father God how we should speak to the situation. In healing we should know what the will of Jesus is, what he said he came to do, and be aware that his words from the cross mean that he has done it. Standing up in front of other people can be a scary place. Jesus let all those present know that he was commanding the 'impossible' to happen.

Lazarus came out alive. How? I try to picture how Lazarus, wrapped tightly in grave clothes, managed to stand up. When he was on his feet did he hop out of the cave? Did he waddle out? How did he come out with his legs bound together? Jesus ordered them to unbind him. Lazarus could not do this for himself, his hands were tied. Someone else had to take the risk of the stench and the infection and what they might see. This is what the healing ministry is about. The medical world is not a neat, tidy, sanitary business, as any nurse or doctor could tell you —nor is the spiritual realm. But this is what he is asking us to do in this ministry: unwind them, unwrap them. That is what we are here for in this ministry —to help unwind, so that they can each deal with their 'stones' with their hands freed and their minds uncluttered, in a safe environment.

In John 11:45 we read, *Therefore many of the Jews who had come to visit Mary, and had seen what Jesus did, put their faith in him.* So they believed *after* they saw it happen. No one's faith was involved in this healing except the faith of Jesus. The disciples had no expectation. Martha, Mary and their friends had no faith or expectation. Lazarus certainly had no faith and expectation; he was dead! The son of the widow and Jairus' daughter were dead, too.

Peter must have remembered the scene, and that of the little girl, very clearly. In Acts 9, when a lovely, kind and charitable lady who was a disciple and highly respected died in Joppa, they sent and asked Peter, who was close by in Lydda, to come. The lady's name was Tabitha (*Gk.* Dorcas). Peter went to the upper room where she lay, and the first thing Peter did was to get all the weeping ladies out of there. The ladies were showing him all the tunics and garments that Tabitha used to make. Tabitha was dead, and they were locked into that death. Jesus had removed from the room all those who were weeping over Jairus' daughter, and those who laughed at the thought that she might be raised to life —and Peter did likewise. Jesus prayed to the Father before he spoke to the situation at the tomb, and Peter did likewise when he knelt by her bed and prayed. Jesus took the hand of the dead little girl and said, *"My child, get up!"* Peter turned to the body and said, *"Tabitha, get up."* Then he gave her his hand and helped her up. So I encourage you if you are sick and have no faith or expectation, or if you feel dead inside. There is life and healing in Jesus. He is the way, the truth and the life.

When people come to the Thursday evening healing services at Beggars Roost, we never lay any burdens of sin or guilt or requirement of faith upon them before we minister healing in the name and authority of Jesus. Jesus didn't. As we have seen in the cases of the dead raised to life, their faith, their sin, their guilt was never at issue. Jesus believed; Peter believed; they had spoken to Father God first. All our ministry team believe. They do not make it incumbent on those who come to the Centre in their sickness to believe. Most people who come are too involved in their sickness to even consider things outside of themselves. In Acts 5:15 we read that *all* who came were healed. It does not say that all who were healed were believers, nor that all who were healed were repentant. All who came were healed. This is our hope and expectation at Beggars Roost. We pray that the day will come, and soon, when all who come to the Centre are healed.

We do not pray *for* the sick. There is not one instance in the New Testament where Jesus prayed *for* the sick. We see many examples in the Scriptures of the different ways that Jesus ministered healing to the sick, such as touching them, speaking to the illness, and even spitting. As part of our teaching course we deal in depth with what we call Jesus' 'models of ministry', and in case studies throughout the book there are examples of some of the different ways of ministering that we have found in Scripture. But any references to prayer are to Father. We talk to Father about what we should do next.

Although I have never seen the dead raised, I have been involved in many occasions where the healing meant the promise of a new life to the sick person. As we noted, Peter, when he raised Dorcas from the dead, followed the model or pattern that he had seen Jesus use, and one of the things I have learned over the years is that there is no set formula for healing —we simply must do what Jesus is directing us to do at the time.

We went to Cramlington

This is the story of how Pat received healing from 'serum negative poly arthritis'. The fact that Pat could not walk on her own and had to be carried into the hall by her friends reminds us of the story of the paralysed man who was lowered through the roof by his friends.

Cramlington is a town in Northumberland some twenty miles north of the Centre. We had been asked to visit an Anglican church plant. It was to be on a Saturday, and the plan was that I would teach in the morning, then after lunch we would hold a healing service followed by ministry with laying on of hands. Members of our team from the Centre were to accompany me, to assist with the time of ministry. In the week before our visit to Cramlington, a well-known British evangelist had been speaking in the region.

Soon after I started teaching in the morning there was something of a commotion at the door as a lady was carried in. This lady spent most of the morning lying on the floor, and all the time I was speaking I just knew in the back of my mind that the first thing that I would be asked to do in the ministry time would be to pray with her. At times like this, even though you know that your trust is in the Lord – and that he has already won the victory, and that you are not the healer, and the responsibility is his and not yours – still the 'buts' and 'what ifs' lurk somewhere in your mind. Teaching time was over, then lunch, then worship, and now came ministry time. The lady was lifted from the floor into a chair for her lunch break. 'That is a bit better,' I think to myself, 'I will not have to get her up from the floor.'

"Randy will you please come over and minister to Pat?" Let Pat speak for herself. She wrote this to me on 1st February 1997:

Dear Randy,
My name is Pat Scovell, I am fifty-five years old and have suffered from serum negative polyarthritis from 11 years onwards.
On Friday 10th January I went to SCC (Sunderland Christian Centre) with friends... to see J John. My friends were excited. I didn't

understand why. I wasn't walking very well. We sang a lot of hymns and J John came on. J John captured my attention – he said Jesus loves us, we sang more hymns and whilst singing Amazing Grace I started crying and couldn't stop. I wanted to say sorry to God for all my sins and asked him to forgive me. I was shouting in my head and I as lifted my head, with my eyes closed a pair of curtains opened and the blackness gave way to fog, fog to mist, mist to light, a beautiful light! I asked God to be in the centre of that glorious light.

J John was asking people to come forward to accept Jesus in their lives. I wanted to go forward but couldn't as all the people around me were on the floor, receiving the Holy Spirit. My friends were dancing and did not realise. After more worship they rejoined us and I asked my friends if someone could talk to me. One came to speak to me; she explained that Jesus had paid for our sins and that Jesus loved me. I recited Romans 10:8–13 to her and we hugged.

The members of our church were acting very strangely, laughing, shouting and dancing. I thought that they looked drunk or mad!

I went to church on Sunday and Caroline and Peter asked me if I would go to St Andrews the next Saturday. I said yes, as it was a healing service.

On Tuesday my left knee was swollen, on Wednesday both knees were very swollen; I had to go to bed as I couldn't walk. I phoned my friend on Friday, explained my problem and she said they would carry me if need be. Bless them!

Randy Vickers told us of his life – healing, really interesting, but I was struggling as it hurt to sit; I couldn't stand and really wanted to lie down. We had a tea break, and I attempted to walk round.

The healing service began; a member of our church got me a comfortable chair and I relaxed into it; we started singing 'Be still for the presence of the Lord is here', and I started crying again and raised my head to the ceiling and raised my arms – my arms started tingling, then electricity flowed up and down my body and LOVE and joy surrounded me – OH SUCH JOY!! Jesus loves me! I started shaking from head to foot, landed on the floor, still shaking in the Holy Spirit!!! God sent a beam of glorious light from heaven over me. He answered my heart's prayer.

Randy came over and asked me to get up. I said I couldn't, I had been run over by a steamroller. Peter and John picked me up. Randy hugged me, and asked me what had happened in my childhood. I explained my Dad had been shot down in the war. I had never really known him. My Mum married again, divorced, married and divorced, married; and my stepfather died of leukaemia.

Randy said did I forgive God for taking my Dad from me? I thought, 'Oh Yes,' and said, 'Yes'! And he asked me to repeat after him, 'Dear Lord, I forgive you for taking my dad from me.' He then felt my hands, elbows, neck. He asked me to turn my neck. I turned it as far as I could; he was praying and feeling my neck. Randy said, 'There's a chap over there with a mustard coloured jumper on, he wants to see you smile.' I turned my neck. I COULD TURN MY NECK. And smiled at the man. He smiled back, encouraging me.

Randy then put his fingers down my spine and onto my hips. I had started shaking again. He sat me on a chair, and felt my knees. Oh I was frightened as they hurt so much! —and said, 'Be gentle'. He said, 'Don't worry,' and it didn't hurt when he put his hands on my knees. In fact it was soothing, and I could feel the heat leaving my knee joints. I was still shaking and he put his hands on my ankles and said, 'Silly girl, your hips aren't in line.' I said, 'Really.' After more shaking, Randy said, 'That's better, they are in line now'!

Randy left me, and two ladies from the church came. One placed their hands on my knees and the other stood behind me and held my hands. I was surrounded by a garland of love. They were so kind and I was crying with joy. Eileen said, 'Right let's bend those knees.'

I said, 'I'll try', and I COULD. I stood up and walked properly, straight up, no stooping, WALKED. Oh thank you, Randy! THANK YOU, GOD. I started shouting for JOY, people were coming over to me and cuddling me. Randy took a photo of me as I was transformed, a different person inside and out.

Randy, the joy and love are continuing, I still find it hard to believe that GOD LOVES ME. I am still walking well! I have spoken in church and told everyone of this miracle, and the Holy Spirit keeps filling me up with such love. I couldn't speak in public before. WITH GOD EVERYTHING IS POSSIBLE. Randy, I hope these words will help someone and that God's healing through you will continue.

Yours in Christ, Patricia Scovell

Pat has continued to go from strength to strength in the Lord. She is a great witness wherever she goes because she wants to tell everyone how much Jesus loves them as he proved his love for her.

What happened that day was following Jesus' commission and

teaching. The day started with proclamation of the good news of Jesus, with teaching about the kingdom being at hand and how we need to be living in the kingdom now. When the ministry time came, Pat was asked to do the impossible. Jesus did this all the time. He told dead Lazarus to come forth; he told the dead girl to arise; he told the dead young man lying in his coffin to get up. He told the paralytic to pick up his bed. He told the man with the withered arm to stretch out his arm. Peter and John told the lame man to get up and walk. All I did was ask a lady to stand up. It was lovely that the two men who collected her that Saturday were actually called Peter and John!

Jesus questioned the father of the epileptic boy about the past (see Mark 9:21). First of all I held Pat in the funnel of his love so that his love and strength and healing could flow into her and she was surrounded by his presence. At the same time I was praying to Father and asking him what to do next. He gave me a cold and desolate image inside myself of a young girl suffering rejection and sorrow. So I asked Pat what happened in her childhood, and out poured this story of rejection and hurt and pain and insecurity. She had had four daddies. Two had died tragically and two had left her before she reached her teens and this awful form of arthritis started to cripple her body. Experience has shown us that arthritic and rheumatic conditions often invade the body through rejection and hurt and subsequent resentment and anger over the situations. Such resentment and anger is not necessarily wilful, nor a cognitive decision. We are hurting. We are in pain. We have no way of alleviating the misery of being left. We know of nothing that we can do to help or put things right again. We are helpless and we do not like it. We feel it must have been something we have done, and blame and resent ourselves. They left us so they must not like us, and we do not like that and resent it. Where is God in all of this? We think he has left us too. All kinds of thoughts, feelings and emotions fill us and twist us. Our spirits have been taking the brunt of the trauma and shock. The body reflects what is happening in the spirit.

As I held Pat, the love of Jesus poured into her spirit, and remember Pat was now born again and the Holy Spirit could minister directly to her spirit. The trauma and the shock were released. The fragmented young part of Pat was being integrated with the adult fifty-five year-old woman. Now I needed her to be completely clear so that this arthritis would have no excuse to return. So I ensured that Pat verbally and mentally was able to forgive her daddies for leaving her, and 'forgive' Father God for allowing this to happen to her. What I mean by this expression, and what it does not mean, is set out more fully on page 126 below. For now we simply note that I do not of course mean by it that God is any sense to blame. I have found that, although we might not consciously have blamed God for all the awful things that have happened to us, or the people we love, we so often have asked him why this should happen to us; how could he allow these things to befall us? Whichever way we say it, or think it, we mean it. We are basically blaming God. We need to forgive all those we feel have been involved in our hurt and loss and pain. We also need to ask God to forgive us for blaming him. Pat was so filled with God's love and power that she could readily do this from the bottom of her heart. Then I had to let her mind and body know that, as her spirit had been released and made whole, so had her body. This is the part I call, 'making faith work'. It is similar to those events in the Scriptures I have already mentioned where Jesus and the disciples told the people to do things which would have been impossible for them if they were still under the influence of their illness. I started to do a 'complete alignment' on her. This is simply a way to ensure that the whole frame of the person, the skeleton, is brought into alignment. Also, all her joints had been swollen and crippled with the arthritis, so I started moving through them from her hands, up her arms to her elbows, and on to her neck.

Here are the next steps I took:
• When I got to her neck I told her that the man in the yellow jumper was smiling at her. This made her involuntarily turn to look and then she knew that her neck was free.
• I then worked down all the vertebrae in her back, commanding them to come into line as God designed them.
• I commanded that anything damaged should be completely restored, any degeneration to be reversed, so that in bone, tissue, muscle and 'whatever' there would be regeneration.
• I called upon the resurrection power and the surpassing greatness of his power towards us who believe (see Ephesians 1:19) to create again any part that was damaged.
• I commanded inflammation and pain to leave.
• I told the spinal column to be open and clear so that no part of the

nervous system could be trapped.

• I ordered the arteries and veins to be open so that the blood would flow freely bringing life to the whole body, and washing out every last vestige of arthritis, even to every capillary and extremity.

• Then I continued on to the pelvic area, commanding the hips to come into alignment so that nothing of the nervous system going down to the legs should be trapped.

• I asked the Holy Spirit to come, as the oil of anointing, to soak into every muscle and fibre, to coat and sheath the whole nervous system so that there can be no cross wiring.

• Finally, I asked Pat to sit up straight in an upright chair and let me take her ankles. Then I commanded her legs and hips to come into alignment, because they were quite different.

• As her knees were particularly painful, I gently laid my hands on them.

One of the strange things I have found is that although my hands never feel hot the supplicant can usually feel the heat inside and on the hurting area, as the pain and damage are released and healed. The thing I always do next is the 'What can't you do?' part. That is where I encourage the person to do things that were impossible for them before the ministry. Amazingly, they may stretch their arms high in the air, saying, 'I can't lift my arms', or bend and touch their toes as they tell me they cannot bend over!

As Pat's greatest difficulty had been in bending her knees and walking, I got her friends to start exercising her particularly in those areas whilst I moved on to the next person needing ministry. We have a photograph showing Pat victorious that Saturday. From that day on, Pat became an evangelist with her testimony. She will go anywhere in front of anyone and tell how God's love healed her. Some weeks afterwards, she came to Beggars Roost and told us how she had seen angels in her garden whilst she was pegging out the washing on the line to dry. She described how magnificent they were. She had looked down and noticed that they wore nothing on their feet. They poured overwhelming love into and through her.

We went to Ripon, Yorkshire

It is not uncommon to find legs or hips out of alignment, and whenever I hear that someone has lower back pain I make sure that we check out the alignment. Sometimes this has been more eventful than I

WHAT FAITH DOES A DEAD MAN HAVE?

would have wished. One evening I was speaking at an FGB dinner in Ripon. I had mentioned in my testimony about legs coming into line, and this encouraged a gentleman of military bearing to ask for ministry because he suffered from that very problem. I asked him to sit straight up in the chair, and knelt down and took hold of his ankles. It was then that he disclosed to me that one of his thigh bones had been replaced by a steel pin. My faith started to drain out through my knees I knew that God could deal with flesh and bones but I had no experience with steel that I could remember at that time. I continued to kneel and nothing happened: not a tremor in his legs. My nose started to run and I could feel it forming a drip on the end ready to drop. What should I do? —use this as an excuse to put down his legs and take out my handkerchief to wipe my nose? Nobody would think the less of me for that. Do you see how I had switched my attention from the healing to myself? I had to turn all my attention back to Jesus and seek the kingdom. As I did this, his leg started to move into line and the ministry was completed.

We went to Brownsville, Texas

Something rather similar happened on one of our trips to Brownsville in southern Texas. We were ministering in a small Episcopalian church. The first person I was called to minister to was sitting right at the back. It was a man who had one leg longer than the other. Dorothy was leading the worship at the front and we had no ministry team to support us. As I walked to the back of the church the congregation turned to watch, and as I knelt in front of the man my back was to the rest of the people. I held his ankles and commanded his legs and hips to come into line —but nothing happened. Five minutes went past, then ten, and I was beginning to feel desperate. I could imagine all those people getting restless, deciding that this was nonsense and wondering when they could reasonably leave and go home. Dorothy continued to sing and I stayed on my knees in front of the man. Inwardly, in reality, I was on my knees before the Lord. I knelt for twenty long, lonely minutes and nobody moved. Then suddenly, in one swift action, one leg moved about two inches into line with the other. The entire congregation cheered. Then there was no holding back as they came forward and Jesus healed them.

We went to Berlin

On another trip to Berlin, a group of us were having dinner and one of the guests was a Catholic lady. During a ministry session after a church service that morning one of the healings had been an alignment of someone's leg, and this was being discussed over the meal. On hearing this, the lady told us that on the previous Friday, just two days before, her doctor had diagnosed her as having one leg longer than the other. She then proceeded to tell us the most horrific story of her life. As a child, terrorists had burst into her bedroom where she slept with her nurse, and they had raped and stabbed her nurse to death. Her father was an expatriate and when he returned to his home country he took her with him, but she was rejected and badly treated by his family. As soon as she could, she married to get away from home. She did not marry for love, but to escape. The marriage went badly and her husband mistreated her. When she was able to leave she came to Germany.

I invited her to come to the dinner at which I would be speaking and ministering on the following night. I knelt in front of her and took her ankles. She was a devout Catholic and took little encouraging to forgive the terrorists, to forgive her father and his family, and to forgive her husband. She was able to ask God to forgive her for marrying for the wrong reasons, and for the hurt she had caused her husband. She asked forgiveness for the things that she had done which had added to the breakdown of the marriage.

When I suggested that she 'forgive God' she hesitated. God was God she said, so how could she? I asked whether, with the all the horrific events in her life, she had she never cried out to God and asked him what he was doing, or where he was, in all the hurt and pain, and ask why this should happen to her. Still she hesitated. Happily, she had brought with her that night her parish priest who was her friend. She looked up to him and he nodded and told her to go ahead, that it was in order. At this she forgave God for all the hurt in her life and asked him to forgive her for questioning. As she did this, her leg moved into line and she was healed.

4

THE ANOINTING BREAKS
THE YOKE

Jesus said to the man with the withered hand, *"Stretch out your hand."* He stretched it out, and his hand was completely restored (See Mark 3:5).

We went to Brownsville, Texas
Back in 1984 Dorothy and I went to visit our middle son David in Brownsville, Texas. David had completed his degree in theology at Leeds University, and in the summer of 1983 was ready for excitement, travel and adventure. Before starting in the world of work he wanted to marry this desire for adventure with giving a year out to the Lord. David had applied to work with the Mission to Seamen and he was assigned to a post in the Port of Brownsville, on the Gulf of Mexico.

At the age of thirteen, back in 1975, without any help or guidance from his parents, David had asked Jesus to be Lord in his life. With no encouragement from us, he had taken himself off to confirmation classes at our local Anglican church. On Sundays, whilst his pagan parents stayed in bed, he would get up and go to church. Little did we suspect at the time that he was praying for us. Not that we would have considered it a dangerous thing for him to do. We did not know then, how powerful are the prayers of children. Within three months of David starting to pray, Dorothy and I committed our lives to the Lord, and shortly after this we were baptised in the Holy Spirit. David was responsible for leading his younger brother Paul to the Lord soon afterwards.

So here was David, deep in the south of Texas, and his mother wanted to see how her child (by this time he was a man of 21, but still her child) was doing. Dorothy and I had never visited the USA so this was going to be a first for us.

On Sunday mornings in Brownsville, David was a reader at the Episcopalian church. On Sunday evenings he was a regular member of the congregation at the Church of the Good Shepherd. This was an independent charismatic church, pastored by Shirley and Gayle Gardner. We arrived about a week before Easter.

The Episcopal church was in interregnum, but I was welcomed and invited to lead services through Holy Week —leading from the praise of Palm Sunday, through the sorrow in the garden of Gethsemane, and the awful bleakness of the cross, to the joy of the resurrection. This was wonderful preparation for the miracles, signs and wonders which God manifested at the Church of the Good Shepherd on Easter Sunday night.

The worship was truly anointed, and when I stood to speak it was into a lake of God's grace and faith. This was one of those occasions when I was excited to hear what I was preaching. The word just poured out. I cannot remember what it was I preached on. Prior to our coming to the meeting the Lord had given me a number of words of knowledge: about a scalp that itched, seven people who were deaf, a stiff leg, and a number of others. Such was the depth of faith, nurtured in the people by Pastor Gayle, that no sooner had I spoken out the words of knowledge than people responded, the itchy scalp leading the way. A teenager came forward, who had injured his knee and could not bend it. This was extremely restricting for a young man who was a keen sportsman. He was so open to receive that within minutes we were running up the aisle together, his knee joint performing perfectly and without pain. Then I was led to the front pew where a tiny, elderly looking lady was sitting. As she lifted her arm I could see that her right hand was completely withered and deformed. Her hand was tightly folded across the palm, so that the fingers touched the wrist. I asked her to stretch out her hand. As I took hold of it, her hand unfolded and straightened, like a closed flower bud opening in the morning sunlight. At first it kept twisting back against the wrist, but gradually it lay open and calm in my palm. It was then pointed out to me that her legs were withered and the muscles on them hardly existed. Normal walking was impossible. She could only shuffle.

She had been like this since birth. I took her arms and helped her to stand, and I spoke to her legs in the authority of the name of Jesus, telling them to strengthen and walk. Dorothy leaned over and told me to take her for a walk of faith. We slowly started up the long aisle together at snail's pace, but gradually gained momentum. When we turned at the top of the aisle I started to skip back down it, and she imitated my actions, and soon we were skipping gleefully together. She could walk. All her movement was restored but we did not see, at that time, any particular restoration of the withered muscles.

A baby was brought to me who had not been able to suckle from her mother's breast or take milk. Her father, who held her, showed me that he had a TB lump on his elbow. The lump disappeared. The mother took the baby away, only to return before the end of the service to say that she had been able to feed the baby naturally.

A number of people declared that they had been deaf and now could hear. We counted them up and found that there were five. At this point, a lady piped up to say that as she had forgotten to bring her hearing aid she had not heard the words of knowledge, but now realised she could hear. A member of the congregation directed my attention to another lady who was still profoundly deaf —she was the seventh. I laid hands over her ears but still she was not healed, and I asked the Lord what to do next. The sense of the words from Romans 10:17 came to mind, ...*faith comes from hearing the message, and the message is heard through the word of Christ.* Who better to know the right words of Christ for this situation, I thought, than the Holy Spirit? I prayed in tongues into the lady's ear and, hallelujah, her ear opened and she could hear. One of the deaf people healed was the father of the baby who had already seen his TB lump disappear!

I cannot remember all the other wonderful healings and signs and wonders that the Lord manifested that night, but there was one sign which I think was especially for me, to help save me from becoming proud and accepting that any of these miraculous things had anything to do with any power of my own. In case I thought that I had preached so well, so moving the faith of the people that they could receive their healing, the Lord quickly pointed out the reverse. Dorothy brought the sister of the lady whose withered arm and leg had been healed, to speak with me. Dorothy said that this lady had told her that her sister had turned to her when I had finished my sermon and asked in Spanish, "What does the man say?"

Her sister had told Dorothy in strongly Spanish accented English, "I say to her, the man say, if you want your healing then come and get it." So her sister had done so. I then found that the majority of the congregation spoke only Spanish and understood no English! That wonderful sermon, those encouraging words of knowledge— 80% of the people had not understood a word, but God in his awesome power is not restricted by the limitations of those who want to serve him.

One morning, four years later, Dorothy and I revisited the Church of the Good Shepherd. A Mexican lady who looked around forty years of age opened the door for us. She greeted us pleasantly in good English and invited us in. We said that we were visiting from England and wanted to see Pastor Gayle. As she ushered us towards his office she told us that they had had a young Englishman called David who used to worship at their church, and that her withered hand and legs had been healed when David's father had come to speak. Dorothy assured her that David was our son. I was delighted to hear her protest that I was much too young to be David's father, but she readily accepted our relationship. Dorothy and I stared at her almost with disbelief. We had thought that the lady who was healed was at least in her sixties, and could not possibly be this sprightly, youngish looking person. She held out her hand to us. This now seemed to be perfectly formed, showing no inclination to curl over into a clenched fist. However, Pastor Gayle, in giving his permission to use his name, told me that it is still not quite normal. The muscles on her legs seemed to be perfectly formed, and all traces of having been withered since birth were completely eradicated. She told us that after she was healed her wish had been to serve as doorkeeper to the Lord in his church. Pastor Gayle had allowed her to do just that, and it was also her joy to be the cleaner of his house.

Further confirmation of the wonders of that first Sunday night was brought to us when Gayle invited me to preach again during that second visit. When the time came for ministry a man came forward. He told me that it was his baby who had been healed —and had never looked back. The baby had continued to be able to feed, and grew well and healthily. He told me that his TB lump never reappeared and that his deafness had gone for good. "But," he said, "when I could hear, I found that I then had tinnitus, which is most irritating. Could the Lord please heal me of that?" So the Lord did.

The anointing breaks the yoke

Generally in the ministry of healing, the role and place of the human spirit has largely been overlooked. Most books on healing deal with healing of the mind, healing of the body or healing of the soul. Even the majority of the books dealing with 'inner healing' and 'emotional wholeness' seldom bring the human spirit into the equation, yet we need to understand that we are 'spirit living a human existence' rather than 'human seeking a spiritual experience'. Whether or not we are born again, we humans have a spirit. God intended us to be in unity and communion with him. Then, at the Fall, this unity and communication with Father God was cut off; it died. Man still had a spirit but it was dead to the things of God. Then Jesus came as man to restore the possibility of that unity and communication.

I want this to be a very practical section of the book. I want us all to know and experience the fact that we can be living under the anointing, and need to do so. I want to see the manifestation of Christ working in and through all who believe. On the first occasion Dorothy and I led a mission in St John the Divine Episcopal Church, in Houston, Texas, I talked about the anointing. We called the weekend 'Cry Freedom', and we saw people set free from some of the raw, desolate places in which they had been living. The second time that we visited, our theme was 'Living in the Kingdom'. We talked about who we are in Christ Jesus, and how the kingdom is not just a life after death experience, not just something of the age to come; rather, for all who believe and are called by his name, the kingdom is now. We saw that through the fact that Jesus was born of Mary. He was fully human. He was still fully divine but, as we learn from the Scriptures, he had emptied himself. It is after his baptism, at which the Holy Spirit descended on him like a dove (see Luke 3:21), that we begin to see his power to heal; now his divine, miracle-working power was manifested. The power to heal which we see in him is the same power that he wants us to have, and which we receive when we have been baptised in the Holy Spirit.

In Ephesians 1:18, Paul prayed that God would enlighten the eyes of his reader's heart, that we might know, amongst other wonderful things, *his incomparably great power for us who believe*. Will you start to let that be the living word within you? Start to pray that scripture into yourself: *God, open the eyes of my heart, that I might know your incomparably great power for us who believe*. That power of which Paul wrote can become something we experience throughout our everyday life.

I implore you to be willing to give up all the intellectual control that your mind wants to hold on to because it makes you feel safer, and remember that Jesus always intercedes for those who come to God through him. (See Hebrews 7:25.)

Jeremiah wrote, *When your words came, I ate them; they were my joy and my heart's delight, for I bear your name, O LORD God Almighty* (15:16). The idea is that we will have the truth, the reality of the word, as our staple diet —every day, for breakfast, lunch, tea, dinner and supper, not just a Sunday morning snack! His 'incomparably great power for us who believe' —Who are those who 'believe'? Those who are born again are believers. Jesus said *...you must be born again* (John 3:7). The new birth is a miracle that happens when we acknowledge Jesus as our only Saviour, repenting of sin, accepting his saving death on the cross of Calvary, and ask him to be Lord in our life to reign in our heart. When we do this personally, we know the truth of John 1:12, *Yet to all who received him, to those who believed in his name, he gave the right to become children of God.* What happens then? Our spirit is reconnected. Our spirit is restored in the communication with God and the things of God, through the power of the Holy Spirit. Then, as Jesus promised, we have eternal life. It is not that we will have it sometime in the future —we have it now. When we are born again we immediately start living in the eternal life of the kingdom. This is the first major difference between those who believe and those who are not born again. Everyone has a spirit, even those who do not believe, whether atheist, agnostic, pagan, all those faiths which do not accept Jesus as Lord. But their spirits are separated from God. They are dead to the things of God.

Jesus spoke of those who do not hear his word: *Why is my language not clear to you? Because you are unable to hear what I say. You belong to your father, the devil, and you want to carry out your father's desire. He was a murderer from the beginning, not holding to the truth, for there is no truth in him. When he lies, he speaks his native language, for he is a liar and the father of lies* (John 8:43f). (See also Acts 13:10; 1 John 3:10; Matthew 13:38.)

You need to know for certain, beyond all doubt, that you have been born again. Death holds no fear for those who have been born again because they are going to go straight to heaven when they die. Seldom do I ask anyone whether he or she is a Christian. Many English people, unless they are of some other definite faith group, automatically class themselves as being Christian. I usually just ask people whether or not they know that they are going to heaven when they die. So often the reply comes back as: 'Well, I hope so', or, 'I am working at it.' They do not understand the biblical promises that mean those who are born again have eternal life and do not come under condemnation. As Paul puts it, speaking to believers of the last day, *we will all be changed ... in the twinkling of an eye.* (See 1 Corinthians 15:52.) Isn't that a marvellous thought? And in Revelation 3:21, the risen Jesus said, *To him who overcomes, I will give the right to sit with me on my throne, just as I overcame and sat down with my Father on his throne.*

If you are uncertain about your future, why not take the opportunity to make it certain today? Pause for a moment now. Ask Father God to forgive you for all you have done that has kept you separated from him. That can include many things, and as I have explained, there is a basic separation from God which applies to everyone who has ever lived, except Jesus himself. And we all have particular sins of which we need to repent. Among the many barriers that may come to mind now, you might be aware of anything to do with the occult or involvement in secret societies. By the occult I include things which may seem trivial to you, such as reading your horoscope or having your fortune told. Whatever sins come to mind (and of course it is impossible consciously to remember them all), thank God for sending his son Jesus to die on the cross that you might be washed clean by his precious blood shed for you. Thank Jesus for loving you and wanting you so much that he was willing to give up his life for you. Then, again in your own words, say something like, *Jesus I surrender my life to you and ask you to come into my heart and be Lord in my life. Thank you Jesus. I receive you as my Lord and Saviour. Now I know I am born again; I have eternal life; I am a son* of God. I tell you, Satan, that you no longer have any authority in my life, and I break all the yoke of your oppression.* (*Male or female, we can still say 'son', because it concerns coming into inheritance.)

The wonderful thing is that that is just the start. Let us now look at the anointing. Jesus lived for about thirty years, so we are told, before he entered into his ministry. We have already noticed that no miracles or healings at his hands are reported until the Holy Spirit comes upon him at the Jordan, following his baptism in water. Many people seem to consider that baptism in the Holy Spirit is a figment of the charismatic or Pentecostal imagination, but in Luke 3:16 John the Baptist proclaims that Jesus *will baptise you with the Holy Spirit and with fire.* Luke 4:1 then reports that Jesus, full of the Holy Spirit, returned from the Jordan and was then led by the Spirit into the wilderness where he faced forty days of testing and temptation, after which he returned to Galilee in the power of the Spirit. (See v. 14.) Jesus went directly to the synagogue in Nazareth where he had been brought up, and quoted from Isaiah as we read in Luke 4:18f.

> *"The Spirit of the Lord is on me,*
> *because he has anointed me*
> *to preach good news to the poor.*
> *He has sent me to proclaim freedom for the prisoners*
> *and recovery of sight for the blind,*
> *to release the oppressed,*
> *to proclaim the year of the Lord's favor."*

For the first time in the Bible, we are shown a vital connection. What is revealed is the work of the Holy Spirit, who we are told, *descended upon* Jesus (3:22), who is now *full* of the Holy Spirit (4:1) and in whose *power* he returned to Galilee (4:14), and then made that declaration in his quotation from Isaiah, which included the affirmation that he (Jesus) was now anointed to preach and heal. As we saw earlier, we need the baptism in the Holy Spirit, and that is necessary for us to minister and heal, under the anointing.

Jesus went from Nazareth, where they would not accept him, to Capernaum, where he taught with authority, healed the sick and cast out unclean spirits. We recall Mark 16:15f as well as the 'commissioning' passages elsewhere in the Gospels that he wants us to do likewise.

In Acts 1, Jesus commanded the disciples not to leave Jerusalem but to wait for what the Father had promised. The promise of the Father was baptism with the Holy Spirit. He told them they would receive power when the Holy Spirit had come upon them. Jesus could not give them the Holy Spirit before this. First, he was to ascend, to sit at the right hand of the Father. We are told in John 7:39, *By this he meant the Spirit, whom those who believed in him were later to receive. Up to that time the Spirit had not been given, since Jesus had not yet been glorified.*

Through the ministry of Smith Wigglesworth, the Lord wrought many miracles on both sides of the Atlantic Ocean, including I believe, some 28 recorded events of people being raised from the dead. Wigglesworth believed that Jesus wants all who are saved to receive power from on high: power to witness; power to act; power to live; power to show forth divine manifestations. I agree with Wigglesworth— Jesus prophesied that anyone who has faith in him will do *even greater things* (than the miracles he did). (See John 14:12). So if you are not sure whether you have been baptised in the Holy Spirit, I suggest you take this opportunity to receive the anointing from on high. Like the apostles in Acts, you too can receive the promise of the Father to be clothed in the power of the Spirit of God. Jesus was full of the Holy Spirit and the power he imparts, and that is what we need. If you already know the anointing in your life, be refreshed, go on being filled by the Holy Spirit, as we are told to do. I am not saying that the Holy Spirit was not already at work in you. A person cannot become a Christian without the Holy Spirit being present in them. The Holy Spirit is already at work. The Holy Spirit descending upon Jesus like a dove at his baptism, like any divine 'coming' does not mean that he was not there before, but that he was coming in a new way. It is evident from Acts 8 that baptism in the Holy Spirit is something more than baptism in water in Jesus' name. *When they arrived, they prayed for them that they might receive the Holy Spirit, because the Holy Spirit had not yet come upon any of them; they had simply been baptized into the name of the Lord Jesus* (Acts 8:15f). The people concerned were baptised Christians but Peter and John were of the opinion that they had not yet received the Holy Spirit.

One of the marks of the Holy Spirit's work in us is that we are open to the hope of the riches and the power which is our inheritance in Christ Jesus. We are open to what he can do for us. The power that is released by the Spirit in the church is the same power that raised Jesus from the dead.

It was years before I fully appreciated why we needed the anointing. From about 1980 I have used different programmes to help me read through the Bible once every year. There is a passage from Isaiah, which I therefore must have read at least 21 times without realising the importance of it until this one time. I suppose part of the reason I had not realised the full implication before was because the translations that I usually read do not use the same language as the Authorized Version, which produces the impact that it was really meant to have on people's lives. On that 21st time of reading it, I knew it was for us today. Isaiah 10:27 tells us that the yoke will be destroyed because of the anointing. The word *shemen* is used 190 times in the Bible and signifies grease, liquid, olive oil, the anointing oil. In translations which use the word 'fatness', this is speaking metaphorically of a fat bull, which has grown so strong it has broken away from its yoke. No longer does it have to go round and round, yoked to the treadmill, it breaks free. Now that is power —power to break the yoke. The anointing is power from on high.

Today we can have all kinds of yokes broken that are binding us to things from which we need to be set free. What is your yoke? It can be: sickness, depression, poverty, spiritual blindness, bitterness, rejection, loneliness, grief. The word says that the yoke shall be broken because of the anointing.

I prefer to pray with people, to minister to people, at a meeting or service when as many believers as possible are gathered together, rather than on their own. People phone us at Beggars Roost and ask whether they can come and see us privately, or better still come and visit them at their home. We normally suggest that they come to a Thursday evening service first, and that we shall start from there, because often what might take weeks or months of private counselling, God can do in a few minutes at a meeting of Christians. Remember when the church met in Mary's house to pray for Peter to be released from prison, something way beyond their wildest imaginings happened. The angel released Peter.

Amazing things often happen when Christians gather at conferences, rallies and events that centre on the good news of Jesus Christ, where there is openness to the work of the Holy Spirit. Is that why so many wonderful manifestations are continuing at so many large events today, in so many ministries around the world? We usually refuse to make individual house calls unless there is a very compelling reason. The healings that I have seen when I have gone out to someone's home have been few compared to when the people come to a meeting. When people come to a service not only is there a combined anointing, but in the very act of coming to the meeting they are already starting to move into their healing. This is why at meetings, rather than go to the people in their seats, we encourage them to come forward for ministry. When they get up off their seats, sometimes very reluctantly, they are giving up some of themselves and moving into the healing that Jesus has for them.

At his rallies Billy Graham always invited those who wanted to give their lives to Jesus to come forward. I am sure that they could all have accepted Jesus where they stood on the terraces, but I feel that Billy Graham knew that the the coming forward was significant as the anointing that would break Satan's yoke off their necks was at work. So often, the moving forward was not just from their seats, but from the old worldly mindset. People excuse themselves from coming to the Centre or coming forward from their seats because they are too shy. My initial tendency was to feel sorry for them, to go out of my way to accommodate them, and endeavour to save them embarrassment. My experience has been that when I did that, immediate manifestations of healing or deliverance or salvation have been few, especially compared to what we see at healing services. It dawned on me one day that, in this context, shyness can be a sin. That may seem a harsh thing to say, but I do so advisedly. Think about it: we are exhorted in the Bible to seek first the kingdom of heaven; to keep our eyes fixed on Jesus. During the plague of serpents in the desert, the Israelites had to look up to the bronze serpent on the pole. They had to look up to God, not at the circumstances surrounding them. They had to trust God to deal with the circumstances whilst they kept their eyes on him. So shyness in this respect is not being humble or self-effacing. It is having my eyes firmly fixed on myself, on how I feel, rather than my eyes being fixed only on Jesus. This kind of shyness is about being fearful of coming into a room where people are. It is about not getting up from my seat and going forward because I am fearful that everyone will be looking at me. It is about *me*. This kind of shyness is a warped pride. Why should we think that everybody would be looking at us? The other people have their own issues to contend with. Jesus' teaching shows us that fear itself is a sin. It reveals all the areas within us where we do not trust him. *Don't be afraid* (Matthew 10:31). *God did not give us a spirit of timidity...* (2 Timothy 1:7). Being fearful of people is allowing ourselves to be dominated by circumstances.

At an FGBMFI conference the speaker was Chinese. He was saying how keeping face was one of the big problems for Chinese Christians. I know personally that 'face' is important to the Chinese because over the years I have had many business dealings with Chinese suppliers. I found very early on in my career that if I wanted to tell a supplier his goods were not up to the standard that we had agreed, I had to be very careful in how my complaint was worded, so that he or she would not lose face and I would not lose his business. My Chinese brother said that Chinese Christians were reluctant to tell colleagues, who were probably Buddhist, about Jesus. Some were afraid to have it known in the workplace that they were Christian because they might lose face with their colleagues and with their family. But my Chinese brother went on to say that if we have been crucified with Christ then we have no face to lose. We are then in Christ and he in us, so we should not be presenting our face but his —and he has no fear of what other people might think.

The doors of the kingdom are open. Come into the anointing of the power from on high! If you have already prayed to ask Jesus to be Lord of your life, I invite you to pray now to ask him to fill you with the Holy Spirit. You could use these words:

Father God, I thank you that you sent your Son, my Lord Jesus, to die for me on the cross so that I might be washed clean of all my sin and born again. I thank you Lord Jesus that you loved me so much you were willing to die for me. Father, I thank you that Jesus rose again from the dead and ascended into heaven, and that you pour out the promised Holy Spirit upon your people. I ask you now, Lord Jesus, to take me and baptise me in your Holy Spirit; clothe me with your Spirit; fill me with your Spirit, empower with your Spirit. I ask you, Holy Spirit, as Jesus promised, come upon me now, fall upon me now, so that the anointing will be upon me to preach the gospel, proclaim that the kingdom is at hand, and heal the sick. I receive you, Holy Spirit.

Now ask the Holy Spirit which yokes are oppressing you and keeping you in subjection to sickness. As the Holy Spirit highlights them within you, using the power of the anointing that is on you and within, you are to command these things to be broken from you. Claiming the protection of the blood of Jesus, declare that the power of Satan over your life is broken. Satan is the thief and liar who wants to rob you. Break any yoke he has over you. When you do,

and arrangements to get y'all down to Laredo, while I was very supportive, when she actually succeeded, I was a good bit scared that these 'weird' people were coming to stay in my house while speaking at our church! Would you be speaking in tongues around me? Laying hands on me? Uh, maybe you'd like staying at the historic La Pasada Hotel instead?

Of course you guys are very normal. After playing a round of golf with you, you quickly (and often) demonstrated that you had no magical powers personally. So the Spirit that joined us in the church the night of your teaching was impossible to contrive and could have only been the true Spirit of God in our presence. Later, the Presbyterians from down the street, who were present at the Episcopal church that night, knew nothing about how it happened, but they knew exactly Who happened. They asked for more of your teachings at their church the next night (ruining our rodeo plans, remember?) A night time meeting at my house manifested more laying of hands, speaking (and singing) in tongues and slaying in the Spirit right in my living room (just what I had earlier feared, and now embraced) from people of both churches. It all seemed quite normal, because God was quite obviously in charge.

During the home meeting gathering of the Episcopalians and Presbyterians, this the last of three meetings, Randy asked me to receive God's Spirit. First to pray for 'a gift' from God personally, where I promptly obeyed by asking for the healing of my daughter. Randy would have none of that, he reminded me and 'forced' me to pray for myself — something I don't remember ever doing in honest fashion. I thought about how my back ached to the point I almost missed playing golf with Randy the day before. I mustered a quiet prayer to God that went something like: "God, I have seen you move and I have seen others touched, yet creeping doubts about the authenticity of the past two days continue to creep into my mind. God, if you are here and if you are real, I pray that you heal my back from the lower back pain I have chronically felt for the past several years. If you can heal my back, I can believe that you are alive and wanting a relationship with me." Afterwards I surrendered to the Spirit and lay on the floor 'slain' in his presence.

A day later I felt better, two days later I had no pain in my back for the first time in years, God showed me he was real and wanting relationship — it was my turn to hold up my part of the deal. If God was telling me yes he IS real (instead of my previous belief that he WAS real), then I needed to know more about him. Who was this supernatural Being and why did he want me to get to know him? He was clearly eliciting my response to his truth —I could be faithful to my promise to him, or I could listen to the lies of Satan who kept telling of the coincidental nature of what happened.

I chose [Jesus], and the journey began. I praise God for his love and I thank him constantly for the very attentive ministry of the Vickers and the effect on me and on Laredo. All because you listened to his call to fly all the way to Laredo, Texas for a one-night talk at the Episcopal church and a rodeo that you never saw.

Here are just some of the yokes that we have seen broken on our visits to that city:

A member of the congregation flew her younger brother to Laredo for our visit from the West coast. She was very concerned about him and his lifestyle. Jesus met with him in power that week and the boy surrendered his life. On the Sunday morning we all rejoiced round the pool as he was baptised.

One evening an elderly man in very shabby clothing shuffled to the front of the church. He was in great pain and had great difficulty in walking. The yoke of oppression was lifted from him. He walked confidently from the church that night. He came back the next evening and we found it difficult to recognise this smart man who walked into the room and told us he had walked, I think it was six miles, to get to the church.

Resentment is a yoke that binds

A couple had recently come from another city thousands of miles away to live in Laredo. The wife's hands and her hips were arthritic and she was in pain. The Lord showed me that really she had not wanted to come to live there. It was largely her husband's desire. Although she did want to work for the Lord, she was still holding onto the past and she did not want to walk away from it. As we stood there, she confessed it to her husband who had been totally unaware of the depth of her feelings. As she made the decision to work for the Lord in Laredo and leave the past behind, her hand and her hips were healed.

Another lady at first did not think there was any anger or resentment within her when I told her what the Lord was pointing out to me.

Then the Lord led us to her son and daughter-in-law, and the story came out. The son had remarried and she resented his new wife because she had an extremely good relationship with his first wife and her granddaughter by the first marriage. The lady was actually empathising and taking in all the pain and sorrow for her daughter-in-law. As she was able to start releasing all this and working through it, then the pain and stiffness started to go.

Denominational yokes can bind

I met up with a man who had had a dream sometime before we went to Laredo. This man belonged to a congregation that did not agree with baptism in the Spirit. He had dreamed that he was woken up by a man with white hair who told him that he had to be baptised in the Spirit. He came up for ministry. He was a very big man, between six foot four and six foot six. I led him in a prayer to receive the anointing of the Holy Spirit. We were expecting him to fall backwards under the anointing when, to our great surprise, he suddenly fell flat on his face. He nearly took us to the floor with him. As he lay on the floor I was led to pray into him and then I called for a lady colleague to pray for him. She knelt beside him and prayed in tongues. Only afterwards did we learn the rest of the dream. In the dream he had fallen on his face after the white haired man prayed for him. I had imagined that the white haired man in his dream signified God, but now it appeared that it could have been me. Then, in his dream, a woman had knelt beside him and prayed in tongues, which he understood.

The yoke of death can bind and blind

Scott Edgar and I were working together when three ladies, arms linked together, presented themselves before us. The two ladies on the flanks pronounced, in unison, that they wanted prayer to heal the eyes of their friend, who was blind. They were three very jolly ladies and they said they wanted their friend to get her sight back so that she would be able to drive herself around again and not have to keep bothering them. They said it in such a fun and loving way that it was obvious that she did not bother them at all. I asked whether their blind friend could speak for herself and tell me what she wanted because it was her sight that was lost. She told us that her sight had deteriorated over the past two years. When I asked what had been happening in her life two years ago, she told us about the death of her husband. She had loved him deeply and missed him terribly because he had been the light of her life. They were lovely, Spirit-filled Christian ladies and they listened attentively when I talked about Jesus being the light of the world, and that as Jesus was the light, we should not make any other person the light of our lives. That place was reserved for Jesus and unconsciously, no matter how lovingly she had meant it, she had made an idol of her husband —and Father God had said that, *you shall not make for yourself an idol* (Exodus 20:4). I asked whether she would be able to say sorry to God for doing that, and ask God to forgive her. It may sound strange but even though we know that loved ones do not choose to die and leave us on our own, we often harbour resentment that they left us. We also often rail at God because he let our loved ones die before we think that they should have done. We need to say sorry to God and ask his forgiveness for all of this.

As the tears ran down her cheeks, she said that she could accept all those things and was ready to pray if I would lead her. Therefore, as I always do, I outlined what we would say in the prayers, to make sure that she could agree with them. When leading people in prayer, especially when they are most vulnerable in times of distress, we must be careful not to misuse our position by leading them to say things with which they would not truly agree. Therefore I always tell them first what we are going to say, and make sure that they understand and agree. I asked Scott to lay hands on her eyes whilst we prayed. Scott clamped one very big hand over her eyes and I led her in prayer about the idolatry, forgiving and asking forgiveness. I then pronounced absolution before speaking to her eyes and telling them to be restored.

I asked her what she could see now but at first Scott's hand completely obliterated all sight. I reminded him that until he removed his hand she would not be able to see anything. He did so, and you can imagine the jubilation when she said that she could read the writing on the banner on the wall behind me. The letters on the banner grew even more distinct, so I handed her a Bible, which she was able to read. Her two sisters in the Lord whooped with joy, and the three of them danced. The other two then wanted prayer for themselves and one of the ladies brought up for prayer every member of her family she could find.

Another yoke of blindness broken

This time she came to Beggars Roost, and later wrote this:

You asked me to write about the healing that I received at the Healing Centre. Just over a year ago I came to the Centre, seeking healing for optic neuritis (inflammation of the optic nerve.) My left eye was painful to move and I had poor vision. It was a particular problem as the inflammation was affecting my 'good' eye. My right eye has always had a squint and little vision.

I came to the Centre after my final appointment with the eye specialist. He advised me that my eyesight would not improve much more. I was told that I had a scar on the retina and nothing could be done for this. It was something that I was going to have to live with. After about three visits to the Centre I began to notice an improvement in my sight. Not only that, I was aware of inner spiritual healing. A few months ago I had an eye test by my optician. I wasn't really surprised to be told that there was now no scar on the retina. I suspected that this was so because of the improved sight.

I am so grateful to the Lord and grateful for the prayers said for me. Thank you Randy and Dorothy for your obedience to the Lord by being instruments in his service. Love in Christ.

The yoke of deafness was broken

We were asked to lead a weekend away for a church in Suffolk. It was a very eventful weekend and the Lord was doing some wonderful things in people. On the Sunday morning, a surprising number of the congregation, including some of the older generation, elected to be baptised by full immersion in the sea. Happily from my viewpoint, their own vicar was present on the Sunday and he presided at the baptisms.

Amongst all the bonds that were broken that weekend I particularly remember a very pretty university student who was an extremely good musician. She had had a great problem from birth in regard to her music, in that she was deaf in one ear. The Lord opened her ear that morning so that she could hear perfectly.

The yokes that war can bring were broken when the war veteran came to Beggars Roost

The war veteran was well into his seventies and some friends had brought him to the Centre whilst Dorothy and I were away on holiday.

He was riddled with arthritis. The team had prayed for him during those weeks whilst we were away. The prayers had covered his time as a machine gunner in the war and praying through fears, guilt and forgiveness, etc. On our first night back at the Centre, I asked if I could pray with him, and it took two of us to get him out of his chair and help him shuffle into a suitable spot. I laid hands on his pelvic area, which was the most painful centre of his disability, and started to speak to the condition. Within a short time he was lying on the floor in the Holy Spirit. He lay with the Lord for ten minutes or more. Margot and I helped him to his feet and I started to encourage him to do those things which had previously been impossible for him —such as bending and stretching, and lifting his knees. Soon his brain started catching on to the fact that he was doing these things without pain. I started to march round the room: left, right; left, right —like a man in uniform, and he followed, starting to grin. As Annie and Elke worshipped, we danced to the praise music. The ladies who had brought the old airman to the centre danced with him too. He was delighted, and when he left for home he walked without help. He promised that the next morning he would swing his legs out of bed before his mind tried to tell him that he could not do that.

5

COME, HOLY SPIRIT

...to open eyes that are blind, to free captives from prison and to release from the dungeon those who sit in darkness (Isaiah 42:7).

Power over evil spirits
We went to Zambia and Alex found faith
In June 1994, whilst on a *Sharing of Ministries Abroad* (SOMA) mission to Zambia, we witnessed a mighty move of God's love bringing a young man from darkness into light and life. We had been invited by friends to join a mission going out to Zambia from their diocese, Bath and Wells. The leader of our group was The Reverend John Woolmer.

Prior to our setting out on this venture, Dorothy had attended a day's teaching and ministry led by Anne Watson. Anne had prayed for Dorothy and she had been deeply impacted by the Holy Spirit in a new way which, at that stage, we did not understand. We had not then heard of the move of the Spirit which came to be known as the 'Toronto Blessing'. Before flying off to Zambia, Dorothy prayed for me to receive whatever she had received. At the meetings in Zambia we were awed by the great but gentle power in which the Holy Spirit moved on the people. We saw them saved, healed, delivered and empowered in the Holy Spirit. John Woolmer, in his book *Healing and Deliverance*, referred to the ministry of Dorothy and myself when dealing with large congregations as the 'Come, Holy Spirit' approach. John's observation in the book is that we had far less trouble with evil spirits than was usual, when we ministered this way. This we found to be true. All the information we had been given and videos we had seen before going to Zambia suggested both that during the teaching and services we would have a great deal of disruption and manifestation of evil spirits, and that we would have to contend with a continuous stream of people wanting attention and prayer for healing and deliverance whilst we were endeavouring to teach. By inviting the Holy Spirit to come at the very beginning of a meeting we found that, by and large, we could get through a day with only the odd disturbance, and as you will read later these could be very odd interruptions. Also, in this way, we were able to minister healing and deliverance jointly to the whole congregation, leaving only a comparatively small healing line at the end, when we invited people to come forward for ministry. So we were able to use all the clergy and the local prayer team to minister, rather than have to do it all ourselves.

When we invite the Holy Spirit to come in this way, God does things so much faster, without us getting in the way. For instance, there was an occasion on the Zambian mission when we were scheduled to meet with, teach, and minister to, a branch of the Mothers' Union in a particular township. We were due to be at the hall at about 9 a.m. As we have so often experienced in Africa, time does not necessarily mean the same thing to everyone involved. On this particular day we were two and a half hours late and did not arrive at the designated meeting place until after 11.30 a.m. When we arrived we were informed that our party had been invited to lunch with a very important man of that region, for 12.15 p.m. It was very strongly impressed upon us that this man was so important that, for this appointment, we would have to arrive on time.

I felt terrible because some of these ladies had started out in the middle of the night to walk miles to the town to meet with us at 9 a.m. One wonderful thing about the women of the Mothers' Union in Zambia is that they never miss the opportunity to sing in praise and worship. The most popular Zambian style of worship, if they are not in church as a choir standing or sitting in rows, is to form a circle and slowly dance round and 'sway' to the rhythm of the song. When we arrived there they were moving round in the usual circle, singing songs to the Lord. As we only had about ten to fifteen minutes to greet them and minister, I was praying and asking the Lord for something special. As I said, many had walked miles to get there because they had needs and healing requirements for themselves, their families and friends. So I decided their greater need was to hear directly from the Lord rather than from us and I asked them to stay in the circle and face into the middle, promising that the Lord was going to bring each of them what they needed. I asked them to close their eyes and put out their hands in front of them, as if they were going to receive a gift. Then I asked the Holy Spirit to come. He came with such great sweetness and power. They manifestly began to receive the healing and deliverance they were seeking. Dorothy and I simply walked round the inside of the circle, thanking and blessing the Lord for all he was doing. When we quietly slipped out after fifteen minutes, to go to our next appointment, they were all still transfixed by the Holy Spirit, oblivious to everything that was going on around them. I left feeling certain that each would receive exactly what they had been seeking and praying for when they came.

Generally in Zambia, and probably most of Africa, times of healing and deliverance can be extremely noisy —because of the manifestation of the spirits, and due to the prayer teams and ministers shouting at the spirits. I have noticed that, not just in Africa but in the UK too, there can be a tendency for ministers to shout, or speak very loudly, when involved in deliverance, and in some cases they even argue with whatever entity is supposedly manifesting. Years ago, Dorothy and I realised that, in Jesus, the believer has the authority, and there is no report in the Scriptures of Jesus shouting at times of deliverance. Nor should one accept every apparent manifestation as being an indication of an evil spirit being present. Those ministering need to be working in the power of the Holy Spirit, exercising his gifts of wisdom and discernment. If the Holy Spirit does not lead you to discern the presence of a spirit, then do not rebuke one! Early in our ministry we realised that our role was to rebuke whatever we discerned to be present, or command it to leave, not to argue or converse with it or them.

In Berlin

It was in Germany that Dorothy discovered one of the ways in which we could accomplish this quietly and effectively. We were in the house of a Christian, together with a number of others, to celebrate a birthday. Suddenly, a big American seemed to go berserk. Cups went flying, children went scurrying, and his friends all jumped on him to hold him down. This, we were told, was not an unusual event. We will call him Al (not his real name). Al was shouting loudly. His friends told us that this was an evil spirit in him and they shouted all kinds of things back. As they held Al on the floor, Dorothy went up to him and quietly but authoritatively told Al to open his eyes. She told him that she would not speak to anyone but Al. As she addressed herself only to Al, he opened his eyes. Dorothy commanded him to look at her so that she could clearly see that Al himself was paying attention. In the Scriptures we see that in circumstances such as this Jesus would not allow spirits to speak: *Moreover, demons came out of many people, shouting, "You are the Son of God!" But he rebuked them and would not allow them to speak, because they knew he was the Christ* (Luke 4:41). Dorothy then told Al to come to the surface, be calm and take control, and she 'closed him down' and asked the Holy Spirit to hold him in safety. He quietened right down. A birthday party, with children and families around, was not a suitable time and place for this type of disturbance. His friends were extremely impressed at my little wife dealing with this big American (and the situation) in such a quiet authoritative way.

Back to Zambia

Now we return to Zambia. Father Kapungwe, who is the saintliest man of God I have ever had the pleasure of working with, was our host in the Northern Diocese. He was Archdeacon of the province. Regularly and frequently he visited all the parishes in his archdeaconry, on a bicycle. Small and thin in stature, he exhibited great resolve to pastor those under his care by riding through the bush and forests on dirt roads, crossing rivers, in hot sun and monsoon rain. Yet he asked nothing from us but that we share the blessing of God. He lived in the vicarage in the town of Mansa with his wife Mary, a lovely lady, somewhat younger than him, and the two of their children who were still living at home.

One morning, during breakfast at their home, I was called from the table because a man had cycled about fifteen miles from a village we had visited the previous week. Mary came out and interpreted for me. The man had ridden on his bicycle all that way, starting before dawn, because he knew that there was more that he had to know and experience. He did not know what 'it' was, but simply that he must

78

have it. I laid hands on him, standing in the dirt compound, and asked the Holy Spirit to fill him. His eyes were open all the time but he became completely unaware of our presence, and his eyes and his face shone; pleasure and joy were written large all over his face. Mary and I watched him, not knowing what he was seeing or where he was, mentally and spiritually. His body might have been there in the early morning sun, but his spirit was not. He stood perfectly still in this state for over fifteen minutes, whilst all we could do was stand and wonder at what he was seeing in the Spirit. Gradually he became aware of his physical surroundings and aware of us. He smiled, collected his bicycle, and rode away without saying anything further. Whatever he came for, whatever he expected, he had received and more, and was satisfied and was gone. Mary looked at me and said that she wanted to know what he knew. So we prayed together and the Lord took Mary, in the spirit, to a place I do not think that I have ever been. When she became conscious of her surroundings again, and my presence with her, her eyes glowed and her face shone and she could not find words to describe the experience. I could but wonder that if the Lord had opened her spiritual eyes, like those of Paul, to the third heaven. She now knew the infilling of the Holy Spirit and wanted her family to know, too. Therefore that evening, at tea time, she arranged for her son to have time with us and he received baptism in the Spirit, together with the ability to speak in tongues. This so intrigued Richard, a young man from Bath and Wells who was travelling with us, that he too asked the Lord to fill him with his Spirit.

The next day, we were teaching in the church at Mansa, and even before we started the meeting an elderly priest, suffering severely from arthritic pains, asked for prayer and was released from pain so that he could sit through the day in comfort. During the service in the afternoon, whilst I was leading the congregation in a time of repentance, and deliverance from evil, a lady sitting at the end of one of the pews elevated straight up in the air, turned horizontal whilst still hovering in the air, came to the ground and slithered away up the aisle like a snake. Richard turned to Dorothy with his eyes wide and asked what we were to do. Dorothy replied, "Sit tight, start praying and leave it to Randy." By the authority of Jesus, the lady was released from the bondage and was soon sitting back in her place, continuing with the service.

In one of the parishes which we visited with Father Kapungwe, the priest was under attack from many of the people living in his parish because he was speaking out against the local spiritist healers and practitioners of divination. This was a courageous thing to do because few of the people can afford normal medical attention when they are ill and therefore resort to whatever is available, no matter what the source. During the teaching I was able to show from the Bible how such practices are an abomination to God. When it came to the ministry time, one of those who came forward was a lady who, when the Holy Spirit came upon her, shouted, cursed, and lashed about. It took the priest and a number of others to hold her. She was chattering loudly like a monkey and flapping her elbows. I learnt from her friends that her name was Beauty. Then, as I described in the situation with Dorothy and Al, in the name and authority of our Lord Jesus Christ I quietly insisted on speaking only to Beauty. She was quieted, and then it was possible to deal with the root problems. I discovered that she was a local magician and spiritist healer. This required repentance and forgiveness before deliverance from the animist spirits that were discerned. Obviously this would not have been possible if she had still been shouting and flapping. After we returned to England it was confirmed that she had been set fully free that day, as she subsequently renounced all the practices in which she had been involved, and became a preacher of the gospel in the church.

At one of the towns we visited in the Copper Belt, the church was packed for our day's teaching and ministry. A lady came to me and asked, "Can Anglicans have the Holy Spirit? —Because my friend is a Pentecostal and she says they have the Holy Spirit and not Anglicans." Richard had changed places on our team with Albert, another young churchwarden from Bath and Wells. Albert started the day quite shyly and tentatively, but the power of the Spirit was so strong in the church that day that he was amazed to find himself, without fear, praying for people, using 'tongues', and watching them overcome by the Spirit —something that was completely new in his experience. The anointing of the Holy Spirit was so strong that afternoon that during the ministry time the majority of the congregation was literally out in the Spirit. At the end of the day, the lady who had asked me the question about the Holy Spirit before we started came over to me with her Pentecostal friend. Her friend was moved beyond words and asked if we would please go back to her house for the evening meal because she wanted her pastor to know the mighty way in which the Holy Spirit moved in the Anglican church. The three of us, Dorothy, Albert and I, went for dinner. The pastor was present, watching but saying nothing. Word of all that had gone on in the afternoon had spread quickly. We had hardly started eating before visitors were knocking at the door and coming in. Some wanted healing and some simply wanted more of the Holy Spirit in the same power that was present during the afternoon. Dorothy, Albert and I took it in turns to lay down our plates and lay hands on the guests, and watch as the Holy Spirit overcame them and flooded them. Albert turned to us and said, "So this is what Richard meant when he told me that the most exciting things happen after tea." The lady and her pastor had no doubt that the Holy Spirit has no favourites when it comes to denominations.

After some time in the Northern Diocese we moved south to the Central Diocese. In the car park, when we arrived, we were greeted by a delegation which included a prominent politician and his wife. Although they were not Anglicans, their close friend was the daughter of the Pentecostal lady in the church in the Copper Belt, and by telephone she had urged her daughter and their friends to ensure that they met us and received whatever God had for them. With the bishop's permission we were whisked away immediately to a meeting in their house. I did the teaching outside in the shade of the house, but when it came to ministry time I felt it safer that we should go inside. This was a wise move because no sooner had I asked the Holy Spirit to come than all twenty or so of them fell to the carpet under his anointing. I learned from them afterwards that this was not something they had encountered before. After dinner the evening proceeded just as it had in the town in the Copper Belt, with a steady stream of visitors. Dorothy, Albert and I were getting very tired that evening, when John Woolmer unexpectedly arrived and we turned over to him the task of ministering to all who came.

The bishop assigned Dorothy, John Woolmer and myself to stay with the expatriate priest for Luanshya, Father Simon Farrer. Simon took us to our first venue where we were to teach and then lead a communion service with laying on of hands for healing. John was to lead the first session of the day and the rest of us sat in the pews with the congregation. We had not been sitting long when someone entered the church quietly and spoke to the local parish priest. He indicated that we should accompany the person who had entered. Dorothy, Simon and I left the church and were led to a compound of a village house, which bordered the church land. There were a number of people standing around in the compound, but the most noticeable of all was Alex. To our consternation, Alex was tethered by ropes round his wrists to two of the uprights of the cooking hut. A cooking hut is round. It has no walls, simply a number of upright poles holding a thatched roof over a dirt floor, to give shelter from the sun or rain, for the fire and the cook. Alex was rather dirty, dishevelled and unkempt. As we entered the compound he slid his bonds down the poles to below his knees and looked up at us from between his legs with his backside pointed towards us, just as young children often do. But Alex was not a child. He was then a young man in his late teens. His mother told us that he had been in this state for some years. We never were very sure as to the full facts about the situation. It appeared that when he was at school he had smoked or taken some kind of drugs, turned strange, withdrawn and childlike. Initially he had been taken to hospital, but the hospital had been unable to do anything for him so he came home. He did not speak or communicate with anyone, and he spent his days tied to the poles of the cooking hut, where everyone could see him. They kept him tethered in the compound to stop him wandering off or becoming violent. There was no intimation that he knew Jesus. I do not think that any member of his family was a committed Christian at that time, although on occasions they may have gone to church.

Those present when we met Alex may have expected Dorothy and myself to lay hands heavily on him and immediately commence, with loud, strong, authoritative voices, to cast out all manner of assorted demons. We discerned fear and unlovedness, but nothing more. Our understanding of the story was that Alex's father had abandoned the family when Alex was very young. We were strongly impressed that unlovedness had entered in and started to consume him, until he had finally withdrawn into himself from the world he knew. He no longer wanted to co-operate or have dialogue with the world in which he had to live. I quietly moved over to Alex. He unwound himself from his upside down state, sat on the earthen floor of the open sided hut, and allowed me to sit close to him and hold his hand. Then I was allowed to put my arm around him and hold him. I held him in love in the anointing of the Spirit. As it came time for us to return to the teaching day in the church, Alex stood with me and as I hugged him I felt his arms strongly pressing around me. Soon after we had returned to the church, his grandfather brought Alex in. Alex sat in the pew next to Simon, who held him as I talked to the congregation. I watched Alex lie down and put his head on Simon's lap. I just knew that afternoon that we should make an altar call to invite people to come forward to commit their lives to Jesus. Alex responded. As I prayed with him I had not a clue as to how much, if anything, he understood about what we were doing.

In his book *Miracle at Crowhurst*, Canon George Bennett, writing of his ministry with Downs Syndrome children, tells of how he would take them in his arms with the love of Christ. As he did so they sensed another power about them, and he would silently claim God's will for them. This is very similar to what the Lord showed me about being a funnel of love. As we hold in love, we get this understanding of the pervading, absorbing activity between the healing power of Christ and the whole being of the sufferer. We left Alex that evening, promising to return in two days time.

We returned on the Friday to find that Alex, though still somewhat locked inside himself, no longer needed to be tied to the poles. He was washed and clean, and dressed in clothes suited to his age. His mother said that he was much better but still all we could do was to hold him in God's love. We did promise him that when he decided it was safe to come out into the world we would help him come to visit us in England. However, as again he did not indicate in any way that he appreciated what we were saying, we left, not knowing how much he had comprehended. Three weeks after our return to England we received a letter from Alex, asking us to return to Zambia to get him. I sent a copy of this letter to Father Simon. After kindly visiting Alex, Simon replied to say that, following our visit, Alex had had a brief spell in hospital and was now a charming young man, clothed in his right mind and back at school, continuing his education. All we had had to offer Alex was God's unchanging love.

We return now to the story of the service in the church on the Wednesday afternoon. After leading Alex and others in the prayer to ask Jesus to be Lord in their lives, we celebrated communion, which was followed by a time of ministry with laying on of hands. It is surprising how quickly one forgets all the wondrous things that you see the Lord accomplish during a meeting. I know that Father Simon started that day as a concerned shepherd of his flock, perhaps rightly somewhat sceptical of our ministry, but as the day went on I am sure that his attitude changed. The wife of the priest in charge of the church, though I did not know who she was, brought her baby to the rail for prayer. When you hold a baby and command a blessing it is virtually impossible to recognise any immediate change. But as the ministry continued, the parish priest, the proud father of the baby, interrupted the proceedings. Carrying the baby in his arms, with a massive big white grin right across his face – there was no way that that smile could have been bigger – he announced that for days his baby had been constipated and had not been able to empty his bowels. I cannot remember how many days, but it was a considerable number and the baby had been in danger. However, immediately after I had handed the baby back to his mother, he had filled a nappy. Never have I seen such joy over a dirty nappy! There were many other healings that afternoon as John, Dorothy, Simon and Richard ministered. For example, John Woolmer and Father Simon ministered to a man who was deaf in one ear and after they anointed him he was able to hear perfectly in both.

A postscript about Alex

I continued to keep in contact and help support both Alex and Canon Kapungwe over the years. Alex finished his schooling at Grade 10, I think. His physical health was never very good, and in November 1999 his mother wrote to tell me that he died in hospital on the 14th November. She wrote: 'The last two days, Alex was singing throughout the nights until Sunday.' The last words that he said to her were, 'Mother, I am going.'

A postscript about Cecil and Mary Kapungwe

Cecil retired from ministry, but because of the acute shortage of younger priests in Zambia the bishop soon called him back into service. The AIDS epidemic in Africa is wiping out a whole generation. Cecil accepted a calling to St Matthew's Church, Chibondo, a very remote village, miles away from Mansa, the town in which he had served for many years. We had visited Chibondo on our visit and I remembered how, on the evening we were travelling to the village, we came to a river just as the sun was setting. The only way to cross the river was to use a raft, which was pulled back and forwards across the river by a rope pulley system. Sadly, when we arrived, the raft was drifting out towards the middle of the river. Canon Kapungwe had to wade out into the water in the gathering dark, clamber on to the raft and pull it back to the bank, so that we could drive the car on to it and travel to the other side. To Father Kapungwe this was nothing unusual, in fact it was luxury —normally he would be on his bike or walking.

I remember that over four hundred packed into the church in Chibondo the next day, and the young priest there estimated the crowd that gathered around outside the church was fifteen hundred. Some had walked all night to get there. Many gave their lives to Jesus that day; many were healed; and many were delivered from evil spirits. A letter I received said that, *It should be noted to you that the lady with powerful evil spirits who took most of your time, the evil spirits left her. She declared herself healed just some hours after you left for Luongo Parish.*

Chibondo has no electricity or running water and the villagers are abysmally poor. The church is on a pretty bend in the river, and when we were there the young vicar was in the throes of building a house between the church and the river. Canon Kapungwe and his wife, Mary, gave up the relative comfort of town life to move to a house which was not yet completed. During a heavy rainstorm one day, as they were sitting in the house after lunch, the rain-weakened building collapsed and a heavy beam fell on Mary. Although they were taken to hospital, Mary died.

I arranged for Cecil to come over and stay with us at Beggars Roost for a holiday. It was wonderful to see his surprise and delight at all the modern day conveniences which we take for granted. To witness his childlike approach to escalators, big screen cinemas, and candyfloss at the fair on Newcastle Town Moor, with the gigantic, noisy rides, was a beautiful experience. When he had arrived, all his possessions for the journey were packed into one briefcase. He had no concerns about his luggage being overweight. He asked for little, and was absolutely overcome with delight when we went to the stores and he was allowed to choose some new clothes. Back home in the village, his only transport was a bicycle which the bishop had given him. This was about the only bike in the village and everybody used it, so that now, he told us, it was inoperable. The saddle was worn out and the tyres beyond repair. He went back to Zambia with at least one new saddle, and I was able to get him the new 'green tyres' which do not need an inner tube and therefore cannot be punctured.

In the villages in Zambia, on a good day, we might have all shared a tiny portion of chicken in the stew. So he never tired of going into the supermarket here, just to look at the huge array of food lining the shelves which was available for everybody, not just especially rich people: whole chickens, half chickens, chicken legs, chicken breasts, roast chickens, curried chicken —all laid out side by side. Then Cecil took my breath away and made me feel so very humble. His reaction to all this abundance was not greed or envy, but admiration. "You people are wonderful," he said, "that you are willing to give up all of this and the comforts you have, to come and stay with us and help us in the villages in Zambia where we can offer you nothing."

Cecil's ambition was to set up an orphanage in his home to care for the young children who are being left on their own to fend for themselves as their parents die from AIDS. He went home to Chibondo with over two thousand pounds, which people had given him, secreted away in his clothing so that it would not be stolen from him as he crossed through Zaire on his way from Lusaka to Northern Zambia. He is now foster father to twenty children living in the vicarage.

'Come, Holy Spirit' ministry

Until I read the phrase in John Woolmer's book, I had never consciously thought of our ministry as being of any particular style, but I well remember the first occasion that I heard the phrase 'Come, Holy Spirit' used in the context of ministry. I was a member of a renewal group in the Diocese of St Albans, in Hertfordshire and Bedfordshire. Each eve of Pentecost we used to organise a service in St Albans Abbey and Cathedral. Three thousand souls used to cram in on those occasions. It was tremendous to have so many people freely worshipping the Lord, complete with music, singing, tongues, prophecy and dance. Each year we invited a 'celebrity' speaker, and closed with ministry for healing at various points around the building as the worship continued. Members of the clergy team used to rotate the responsibility each year for the various aspects of organisation. On this particular evening I had organised groups of prayer ministers to be in place, at the various points around the cathedral, when the time for ministry came. After the speaker had finished, Bishop David Pytches was supposed to stand and announce that there would be ministry available at these points, explain where they were, and ask people to make their way to these locations. I was standing in the nave, immediately in front of him, ready to direct people. But Bishop David did not do what we expected. He simply jumped to his feet and said, "Come, Holy Spirit." And come he did, in awesome power. People started falling off the pews. Bodies fell all over the place in the Spirit. Nobody, not even the prayer teams, could make their way to any specific location. So we just started ministering where we stood. Soon I was so completely surrounded by bodies lying in the nave that I was marooned for a while and could not move.

Amongst the many wonderful things God did that night, I particularly remember two. An elderly lady pushed another very elderly lady down the aisle towards me in a wheelchair. I cannot remember what kept her from walking. Nor can I remember what I said, other than telling her to get up. She got up and she pushed the wheelchair back down the aisle. There was a wonderful follow-up to this, which I heard later in the week. A young friend of ours from the Baptist church had brought his father, who was not a believer and was very sceptical, to the cathedral that night. On seeing the lady being pushed up the aisle in the wheelchair, the father decided to follow and see what happened. As he heard whatever the lady and I said, and then saw her stand up and walk, he became a believer. He was baptised in the Baptist church soon afterwards.

I was called to another lady, who had been brought by her friends. The noise in the cathedral was so loud I could not hear what they said. I asked the Lord what to say and subsequently I told the lady that she should forgive her mother. She shook her head, there was nothing to forgive her mother for. Then I told her she had to forgive her grandmother too. The lady replied it was her grandmother's entire fault. I told her that she must forgive them both. She did, and then she gave a loud scream as she raised her right arm in the air. "Look," she said to me. "This thumb has been stiff for eighteen years. I have not been able to move it, but now I can bend it."

So that was my introduction to 'Come, Holy Spirit' ministry, and it was many years before the 'Toronto Blessing'. But there is no doubt that when we returned from Zambia that same anointing was still strongly on us. One Thursday night, soon after we returned, when it came to ministry time at the healing service at Beggars Roost, I simply invited the Holy Spirit to come. Everyone present that night was overwhelmed by the Spirit right where they sat, and there was quite a number because a group had come from an independent church in a local town to see what this was all about. Dorothy and I looked at them and realised there was nothing more for us to do, so we went to the bar and had a cup of coffee and waited until we were needed. I understand that whatever took place changed that church. The senior pastor received an unexpected blessing and a gift of tears. Some of their congregation could not accept the changes and left the church. Some years later, a man who I knew had been one of the elders of that church came to me and apologised and asked forgiveness for the resentment that he had held towards me following all that happened. All I had done was say, 'Come, Holy Spirit.'

The learning process.
When Dorothy and I came to know Jesus personally, we knew of no one around to disciple and teach us more. Our local vicar was a wonderful man, who we came to know and love when we joined his congregation, but his knowledge and understanding of these areas of spirituality was limited. At this stage we did not even know that there were such places as Christian bookshops where you could find books on a wide variety of Christian subjects. It must have been about two years before Dorothy discovered the Christian bookshop in Hitchin. One of the first books I found there, by Roy Jeremiah, told the story of the London Healing Mission. As soon as I could, I paid a visit to 20, Dawson Place. Sadly, I was not able to get down to the meetings there very often, but Dorothy and I became home intercessors for the Mission. Many years later, after Roy died, The Reverend Tom Jewett and his wife, Anne, took over as wardens of the Mission. They became, and still are, very good friends, from whom we have learned a great deal over the years. Tom's book, *The Good News that Nobody Wanted to Know*[1] is the best reference book on the healing ministry that there is, and ought to be on everyone's bookshelf.

When, two or three years after conversion, I joined up with the FGBMFI, I learnt much more through friends and colleagues in that organisation, but for a considerable time we had only the Lord to teach us. I think of John 16:13, *But when he, the Spirit of truth, comes, he will guide you into all truth. He will not speak on his own; he will speak only what he hears, and he will tell you what is yet to come.* And 1 John 2:27, *As for you, the anointing you received from him remains in you, and you do not need anyone to teach you. But as his anointing teaches you about all things and as that anointing is real, not counterfeit—just as it has taught you, remain in him.*

This means what it says. The Holy Spirit teaches us all things necessary, as we are open to him and read the inspired word of God. Paul did not learn what he knew about our Lord from consulting anyone, but directly from the Lord, spending three years in Arabia before his meeting with Peter in Jerusalem. (See Galatians 1:17-19.) I am in no doubt that the Lord taught us what we needed to know.

Knowing versus understanding

I wrote earlier of the human spirit. Consider these words of Paul: *For who among men knows the thoughts of a man except the man's spirit within him? In the same way no one knows the thoughts of God except the Spirit of God* (1 Corinthians 2:11). This is a powerful analogy. Only the Holy Spirit (who is God) knows the thoughts of God; only the human spirit really knows the inward thought of the person. So it is that one of the functions of the human spirit is as the centre of our 'knowing', and we need to learn the distinction between understanding and knowing. The Holy Spirit, knowing the thoughts of God, can transmit these directly to the spirit of man, and thus into the depths of our 'knowing'. Watchman Nee affirmed that the difference between the two words 'knowing' and 'understanding' is incalculable. He says that the spirit knows whilst the mind understands. The Holy Spirit enables the believer's spirit to know, and our spirit instructs our mind as to how to understand these matters. I feel sure that is why so many people have so much trouble in being born again and so many Christians have difficulty with the idea of baptism in the Spirit. Their minds want to understand before they will accept what their spirit already knows. They want first to intellectualise it, filter it and academically explain it. They want a clear and detailed account of the relevant structure surrounding the circumstances before they will accept what the Lord is bringing —that which he can bring to each individual, through the revelation of the Holy Spirit. Recall again Paul's prayer in Ephesians 1:18, *I*

*pray also that the eyes of your heart may be enlightened in order
that you may know the hope to which he has called you, the riches
of his glorious inheritance in the saints.*

So the 'eyes' of our 'heart' or spirit need to be opened. An
intellectual understanding of God can be bypassed, and go straight
into the spirit, so that the person *knows*. Is this not the same way in
which, one night when I was 39 years of age I just *knew* that Jesus
was Lord, even though I had gone to church regularly during my
youth and teens and I had been confirmed? I did not understand it,
but I knew him and came into a relationship with him. Father God,
Son and the Holy Spirit. I had not had one bit of teaching about the
Holy Spirit, but there and then, that night, I *knew* he was a real, live
person. When Colin Urquhart prayed with me, for me to be baptised
in the Holy Spirit, I had no real understanding of what this meant at
the time. I had no emotional feeling about it whatsoever. My body
gave no indication that anything had happened, but I *knew* that Jesus
had baptised me in his Holy Spirit. It was only as the months went by
that my mind and body started to understand what my spirit already
knew. In fact Dorothy and I had already started to move into things
of the anointing and the gifts of the Spirit in prayer and ministry
before my mind started to realise that things were very different and
life was very different. My ways of thinking and 'being me' were
very different.

Introduction to deliverance

I thank the Lord with all my heart that he can and will teach us directly
in this way. Otherwise we would have been completely at a loss when
a Christian friend brought a lady to see us. She introduced her as
being a member of the spiritualist church, who was in depression. The
lady said that she had a spirit of death on her and was terrified. We
asked her why she had come to us and not to members of her own
church. Her reply was that they would not have the power, and
that this needed a Christian to deal with it. Without any previous
teaching on the gift of discernment of evil, having seen something that
looked like a black silverfish sliding across the lady's eye, Dorothy
asked the Holy Spirit what this meant. He revealed that this was the
representation of cunning and deceit, so we knew that there was more
that she was not telling us. As Dorothy rebuked this evil presence
the lady's eyes brightened and were clear.

The lady then told us the full story which included 'astral projection'. She told us how she would meet with another person on the 'astral plane' or by 'telepathic communication'. Although she did not realise at the time that this was wrong, it had finally brought her into deep depression and suicidal feelings.

Over the years in this ministry we have learned that one cannot allow any expression of what you are thinking or feeling to show on your face as you listen. I do not know if we succeeded that day, because this was way beyond anything that I had ever thought possible outside of a Dennis Wheatley novel. I had thought that astral projection was a mythological phenomenon dreamed up by the authors of horror stories, but here, if we were to believe her, was an actual practitioner of this.

We implored her to leave the spiritualist church and give up these assignations, as we could do nothing more about the spirit of death until she repented and asked the Lord to forgive her. She would not do this at that time. She then left.

She returned about two weeks later because she was being tormented by the spirit of death, which would stand at the foot of her bed, and she wanted to be free. So she repented and committed her life to Jesus. We were then able to rebuke the spirit of death and tell it to leave her. In the weeks that followed we could see that she was free. Dorothy took her to the 'Life in the Spirit' seminars, which were being held at the Catholic church. She left the spiritualist church and joined a Christian congregation.

These were years of living in God's grace and covering. This case opens up the debate on whether it is absolutely necessary for a person to have committed their life to Jesus before any form of deliverance should take place. It is well accepted that Satan is a legal expert and therefore only when any sin has been brought under the blood of Christ and there has been forgiveness and repentance has Satan no power or legal right to manifest any sort of influence over a person. Until then any demon which has been delivered from that person can come back. However, might it not be through the ministry of deliverance that the person can be set free to accept Jesus as Lord? Dorothy discerned evil and cunning and rebuked it. With those out of the way the lady was open to be honest with us, culminating in her receiving Jesus into her life and being totally set free from the spirit of death. I think there is much evidence in the Scriptures to support this position. As we see from the models of Jesus and the apostles, deliverance is a normal, everyday part of the Christian healing and wholeness ministry. Seldom in Scripture is there a passage which refers to healing without referring to deliverance. Also, much of the terminology is interchangeable. For example, both Luke and Matthew refer to Simon Peter's mother-in-law being cured of a fever, but, in Luke's Gospel, Jesus rebukes the fever as one would rebuke an evil spirit. Did he see this as being a spirit of fever, without actually using the terminology? If so, how many other references to healing could also be counted as deliverance? *So he bent over her and rebuked the fever, and it left her. She got up at once and began to wait on them* (Luke 4:39). Whereas in Matthew's Gospel Jesus simply touches her and she is healed: *When Jesus came into Peter's house, he saw Peter's mother-in-law lying in bed with a fever. He touched her hand and the fever left her, and she got up and began to wait on him* (Matthew 8:14f).

In Matthew again we see the need for deliverance simply listed as another illness which needed healing: *News about him spread all over Syria, and people brought to him all who were ill with various diseases, those suffering severe pain, the demon-possessed, those having seizures, and the paralyzed, and he healed them* (Matthew 4:24). As the sick were coming from all over Syria, as distinct from Israel, it is probable that many were not even Jewish and had no expectation that he might be the Messiah who was promised. Yet he delivered them. In Matthew 15:21–28 we have the story of the demonised daughter of the Canaanite woman. At first Jesus hesitated, but then, because of the faith in him that he saw in her, he agreed to accede to her wishes and the daughter was healed. In Matthew 8:28–34 we have the story of the demon-possessed men in the country of the Gadarenes. The narrative style, both here and in the Luke story of the man named Legion because of the number of demons involved, would indicate that these men were not men of faith prior to being delivered and set free. Moreover, the evidence of the Luke narrative is that the man named Legion not only became a believer but also an evangelist, following the ministry of deliverance. However, concerning those involved in ministering deliverance, if we have unconfessed and repeated sin in our own lives and have done nothing about it when the Holy Spirit has pointed it out to us, then we are open to trouble. But with a clear conscience before God, and with the authority that Jesus has invested in us, and with the anointing of the Holy Spirit, then we should deal with such things as we meet them. I stress, though, that if we want to be free to do God's will then we have to walk in holiness and righteousness, in the armour of God. Our breastplate is righteousness, which is God's gift to those who believe, but which we have to keep *in place* (as Paul teaches in Ephesians 6:14) —and that implies continuing obedience, and repentance as often as necessary. We have got to know our authority over the powers of darkness, and we cannot be in bondage to them.

Healing or deliverance?

Let me give examples of two very different ways in which two very similar conditions were healed in the same person. The person was my wife, Dorothy, and the two similar conditions were the 'fear of water' and the 'fear of flying'. Both conditions were severe and deep-rooted. With regard to water, Dorothy could not even take a shower because the idea of water on her head was terrifying. With regard to flying, this got worse and worse over a number of years. The last occasion on which I saw her fly before she was healed was a journey back from France to England, on virtually the shortest flight possible, from Le Touquet to the south coast. I was leading a group of salesmen and their wives for a weekend in Paris. Dorothy was attempting to dull the fear within of the flight to come and used a sedative which the doctor had prescribed. When we got on the aeroplane and buckled up, Dorothy fell fast asleep before take-off. But as the plane started down the runway, despite being unconscious to the world around her, the fear was so deep-rooted that she started to cry. The tears rolled down her cheeks as she slept. Dorothy refused to fly after that.

Some years later, after we had come to know Jesus as Lord in our lives, Dorothy taught Sunday school. One Sunday the subject of summer holidays came up and they asked her where she was going. Inadvertently, she revealed that I wanted to take the family to Malta but we could not go because of her fear of flying. "Well Miss," came back the suggestion, "should we pray for you and ask God to take away the fear, and then you can go?" Dorothy demurred but this raised the question of whether she did not believe all the things she had been teaching them. Reluctantly, Dorothy agreed to being prayed for. "Dear God, please take away Miss's fear of flying", or something quite as succinct, was the prayer which was offered. After that, Dorothy felt honour bound to go through with it and we booked the holiday in Malta. The flight was no problem, and since then we have flown long haul and short haul without any difficulty. When she returned to the Sunday school class she expected them to be eager to know about her flying experience. Proudly, she told them that she had flown and not been the least bit frightened, expecting them to be thrilled —but not a bit of it, they had expected nothing less.

When our youngest son Paul was fourteen, and his older brothers were off doing their own thing that summer, I suggested that Paul, Dorothy and I went on a sail training holiday in Salcombe, Devon. Dorothy bravely agreed to this. Her first shock came when we arrived at Blue Water Sailing to find that not only were we to spend the days training in small dinghies on the estuary but that we were also going to sleep on board a boat moored at the jetty. The week went along quite happily because we spent all the time on top of the water and did not have to go in it. However, we all soon knew that on the last day, in order to get our Royal Yachting Association certificate for dinghy sailing, we would have to carry out a difficult manoeuvre which involved getting into the water. It is necessary to show that the candidate can right a capsized dinghy. This has to be done twice, once as crew and once as helmsman. The dinghy is overturned, with both the crew members dropping into the water. They may need to swim under the boat to get into the right position to haul on the sheets to turn the boat upright and then be scooped back in as the mast rises up out of the water. Good co-ordination is needed, as in a two-person dinghy one crew member stands on the centreboard while the other one is scooped up inside the boat and then helps the other back aboard. As the week went by, the horror of this prospect grew larger and larger for Dorothy. Finally came the Friday morning. We donned wetsuits and lifejackets. Dorothy, who could not swim, also had the use of a car tyre inner tube around her. We all sat on the jetty, cheering on each of our fellow candidates as they performed the manoeuvre. Then it came to Dorothy's turn. Clinging tightly to the jetty, she followed Paul into the water. Then she froze and could not swim out to the dinghy. She started to cry and her teeth chattered. All our new friends gathered around, sympathising with her and encouraging her. A young Argentinian lady, who was also a medical doctor, jumped in beside Dorothy to console her. Our ship's skipper and sail trainer was a wonderful gentleman, and a retired naval officer. He said that they all had the utmost admiration for what Dorothy had achieved thus far, and the courage that she had displayed was above and beyond the call of duty. Therefore he kindly suggested it would be no dishonour to leave it at that and climb on to the safety of the jetty. During all of this I had been sitting, praying hard.

Dorothy looked up at me and asked what she should do. I asked her whether she wanted to climb out now and keep her fear of water, or stay in and beat it. The gasps of disbelief and horror that went up from those who until that moment had counted me as a friend had to be heard! They all stared at me, hard and venomously. Dorothy said that she wanted to beat it. Dorothy asked the Lord to forgive her for holding fear. This paved the way for me to start praying aloud to Father God and rebuke in Jesus' name, all the elemental spirits that then came to mind. I have since learned to call that discernment. This went on in complete silence and disbelief from the others until I just knew it was done. Dorothy had stopped crying and shivering. She called to Paul, and they both swam out to the dinghy, climbed in, performed the manoeuvre twice without problem, and, to loud cheers from the crowd on the jetty, swam back to shore. Dorothy was greeted warmly for her heroism. They still looked at me as if I were a rat that should crawl back under a stone!

Dorothy asked me how you get out of a wetsuit, and I told her that I had heard the best way was to stand under a shower and peel it off. So we retired to our cabin and Dorothy stood under the shower with the water cascading down on her head as I helped her peel off the rubber suit. After the holiday had ended, when we returned home, Dorothy signed up for swimming lessons, and one of her greatest treasures is her certificate gained for swimming.

Note
[1] Tom Jewett, *The Good News that Nobody Wanted to Know*, Taswegia Pty. Ltd. ISBN 0 95870 921 1. (Contact details available from The Northumbrian Centre of Prayer for Christian Healing.)

6

PROPHETIC HEALING

Released into joy

"If you are here from God, you tell me what I need prayer for."
Dorothy and I were speaking and ministering at an FGBMFI breakfast
meeting in Berlin. I had asked this very large man what he wanted me
to pray for and that was his reply. He was right. I had been working
on automatic pilot, proclaiming the gospel, laying hands on the sick
and expecting them to be healed, without really paying attention to
Father God. As you can imagine, this big German's reply stopped
me right in my tracks. We need to be listening to Father God at all
times, asking him what he wants to do. Much of the training that we
give to our team at the healing Centre is in the prophetic. This means
listening to God and speaking out what he gives us to say.

When someone comes forward in a time of ministry we ask him or
her what their need is and what they would like us to pray for. If they
tell us what the problem or situation is, we acknowledge that we have
heard and understood by repeating back to them what we understand
they have told us. Part of the healing process for people is to know
that they have been heard. However, even as they approach us we
start asking Father God what he wants to say or what he wants us to
do. If the person has simply come forward asking for prayer and we
do not hear Father say anything to us, then we say nothing to them
and stand with them in silence. I think that this is the hardest thing
for any of us to learn at first. Jesus' ministry of healing is a prophetic
ministry. Jesus only did what he saw the Father do, and said just what

the Father told him to say. (See John 5:19 and 12:49.) Therefore, as Jesus is the healer, we endeavour to follow what he has shown us as the Holy Spirit leads us. Then we speak out what he has told us to say. We do not give our considered opinion of what we think he really means, we speak out what he says and only that. So often it can sound meaningless to us and make no sense at all, but to the petitioner it can make complete sense.

For example, I was praying once with a close friend. Frequently when things got difficult or awkward he would back out of the situation and refuse to take any responsibility. On this occasion we were working in the same ministry group. A fairly strong difference in opinion had arisen between the two of us together on one side and the rest of the team. We two had agreed on what we should say and the action we should take. When the subject came up at a meeting I spoke out as we had discussed, but when they turned to him, he said nothing and left me sitting totally isolated. The two of us met for prayer in the early morning, as was our practice. As we prayed, the Lord showed me a little wooden toy wheelbarrow. It was painted green on the outside and yellow inside. The Lord often speaks to me through pictures. The prophetic is not just about hearing voices. I often speak out aloud when I am talking to God, but I have never heard his voice speaking audibly to me, from outside myself. Some Christians hear the voice of God audibly, and of course this has biblical precedents. We think especially of the Father speaking over Jesus at the baptism in the Jordan. Sometimes I have pictures or impressions, sometimes I see words, or hear words inside myself, or just know the words to say. Sometimes in cases of sickness I feel the pain or hurt in whichever part of the body the person has the problem. On this occasion I described the wheelbarrow. My friend said, "That was mine, and my brother broke it and I got the blame as usual." He then went on to describe how his younger brother was always up to mischief but my friend always got the blame from his mum and dad. His parents expected him to be responsible for his brother and look after him, but always blamed my friend for anything that went wrong. He realised that, all those years before, he had made a decision inside himself never to take responsibility or the blame for anything again, if he could help it. Now we knew how to pray to minister to that young part of him which had been so hurt, so that this part of him could grow into the adult that my friend now was. The Lord showed us to ask for holy boldness. My friend really did grow in holy boldness, and from then on we were able to stand strongly together in many situations. I could have dismissed the idea of a toy wheelbarrow as meaningless imaginings, but have learned not to discount or try and interpret anything that is given to me in prayer.

When ministering at the Centre we might also be led to pray in tongues. But we do not make up nice prayers which make us feel better and hope will make the client feel better, prayers which we hope and feel will be suitable for the occasion or the situation that has been outlined. We will only pray Father God's will. Therefore if their request is for the healing of a physical illness, then as we know it is the nature and will of God to heal, and if he does not give us anything different to say, we can speak appropriately to the sickness and command the body into healing. In chapter three I gave the example of praying for Pat Scovell's physical condition. In Pat's case this was after clearing all the situations of rejection and forgiveness and so on, as Father led me, but if he had not made me aware of those things I could have ministered directly to the physical condition as I described there.

We return to the incident with which we began this chapter —the German man whose comment had put me on the spot. I was frantically asking the Lord for forgiveness for not coming to him first, and asking him what I should do next. Then I had to trust. He does not always explain to me first what I should say and do, so that I can consider it and then consider my alternative courses of action. Sometimes I have to act instinctively, or as I think of it, acting as the Holy Spirit directs my spirit to direct my body, without my mind being involved. I often do not know what I have to say until I hear myself saying it. Instinctively, or perhaps knowing inwardly what I was to do, I put my hand on his chest and started speaking to the problem with his heart. "Yes," he said with great satisfaction. "That is the problem." You can imagine how the rest of the people responded —they all wanted their problems discerned.

I remember that Dorothy called me over to where she was ministering to a lady. She told me that there was a blockage somewhere and asked if I could add anything. Within the hearing of them both I asked whether the lady had told her about the two men with whom she was sleeping. The lady blushed guiltily. As Dorothy told me later, the lady had mentioned one man but not two. When this area of her life was opened up and dealt with appropriately, then the lady was able to appropriate her healing.

To go back to the subject of words of knowledge that appear ridiculous or do not seem to make any sense at all when you receive them, our team has learned not to be embarrassed about them. As with any words of knowledge or prophetic words, one has to offer them and invite the person concerned to consider whether or not they are of any significance to them, and to weigh them or test them carefully. Although we might consider ourselves to be moving in the power of the Holy Spirit, we are still very much of the flesh. We are not infallible and we can get things wrong. We have our own strongholds, which can unfortunately colour what we say and do, even though we may consider ourselves to be very spiritual. We are in fact working in a spiritual dimension, and we always need to have in mind 1 John 4:1, *Dear friends, do not believe every spirit, but test the spirits to see whether they are from God, because many false prophets have gone out into the world.*

I am not saying that people ministering would intentionally or maliciously give false prophecies (although this can occur in some places), but we can all make mistakes. I have heard prophecies from some of the biggest and most respected names which have not been correct. Or, let me say it this way, they have not yet come to fulfilment when the timescale in which they were framed is some twenty to thirty years overdue. I still very much respect those people, because, when weighed alongside the tremendous anointing that has been on them over the years for teaching, healing and evangelising, these errors in prophetic terms seem of little consequence, especially when you consider that in 1 John the onus is put upon the listener to test for himself. So we would give the same admonition about prophetic words as we do with any teaching that Dorothy and I give. We always urge the congregation to test everything we say against the Scriptures, and not just to believe what is said simply because we have said it, and because they like us or respect us.

Asking God for more information

I also learned, very early on, not to just accept that the initial word one receives need necessarily be the sum total of all that God is willing to reveal to us. I remember one night when I was speaking at a meeting in Hitchin. Dorothy and I had moved away from the area some time before, and had been invited to return for that evening. Many at the meeting had known us for years, and Jesus said (in Matthew 13:57) *"Only in his home town and in his own house is a prophet without honour."* To all intents and purposes we were in our home town. I had given out a number of words of knowledge but had no response from the meeting. So I had to go back to Father and ask him for more. One word had been for a person who had an injury and pain in the right cheek. As the Lord revealed more, I spoke it out until the person could not deny to herself that it was her. I was able to say that it was a lady, and the injury was because of an accident; that she had been riding her bicycle and had gone under a tree, and a low branch had hit her in the face.

In another case, I forget what it was the Lord wanted to heal, but I had to keep on giving information until they could not deny it was for them. I was able to tell the meeting that the person had not decided until late in the week that they were going to come. Then I had to go further and mention that, in fact, it was that very afternoon that they made the decision. Still they did not respond. It was only when I added that they had phoned the organiser and had got the very last ticket for the evening that they accepted that God was talking to them and wanted to heal them!

We need to encourage our prayer teams to talk to the Lord about the words that they get, and fill them out, so that there can be little doubt in someone's understanding that God means business for them. This is not to say that a word of knowledge cannot have reference to more than one person. In America recently, before a meeting, we were having a time of prayer with some of their leaders and prayer team. A young lady said that there was someone at the meeting who had a problem with his or her right knee. I stopped her and suggested that such a word could possibly include at least half a dozen people who would be present that day. For a start, I told her that I knew that it concerned a man and not a woman, so asked her what else she could say about him. She was a little taken aback, but prayed for just a second and then said that it was a man and that he was six feet four inches tall. Therefore I was not surprised when during the ministry time a man came up to me and told me that he was six feet four and had a problem with his right knee. The Lord promptly healed it.

'Cry Freedom' in Houston

On the first occasion that we were invited to St John the Divine Episcopal Church in Houston, Texas, by that wonderfully humble man of God The Reverend Dr Laurens Hall, it was suggested that we fly over a couple of days early. This would allow us to meet up with their prayer team and some of the people with whom we would be involved. Dorothy and I replied that we did not want to offend anyone but would prefer not to meet and socialise with any of the people who would attend the conference until after the first sessions on the Friday evening, with the exception of course of J.B. and Ellen Mallay who were to be our hosts. The reason for doing this was because it was our expectation to arrive with words of knowledge and deliver these during the first session. We did not want anyone to be able to suggest that these were based on information that we had been given by people we had met or that we had elicited at the various pre-conference gatherings that the church had wanted to arrange for us. I was so very glad that we did this, for reasons which will become clear. The mission was in the September and I opened the conference with the following introduction:

During July in my morning meditation I was preparing for our visit to Texas and into my mind came the idea that every Monday, Wednesday and Friday in August I should only have bread and water. Being a man I accepted that. When I told Dorothy, being a woman she questioned that. She asked, "Can you have anything on the bread?" When I got to lunchtime on Monday 2nd August I decided that God had not said dry bread so I had low fat spread as well. But as Dorothy will tell you, when we were preparing, although the theme for the mission came readily to mind and the titles for the individual sessions, when it came to writing my material I just could not do it. I have used up days and days of sunny weather, and these can be a precious and rare commodity in England, looking at the titles, reading notes, reading Scripture, listening to others and feeling more and more desperate and hemmed in, wondering what was frightening me. Dorothy suggested that it might be the long list of the names of Doctors of Divinity that adorn the headed notepaper of St John the Divine —that I was being dominated by the idea of being judged by this host of academically accredited theologians. This was very true and I had to repent of it and be set free of domination and fear of man. I was feeling trapped.

On Tuesday 3rd August I opened notes that I had prepared years
ago on the theme 'Freedom' and looked up the Scriptures again.
There, highlighted, jumping off the page at me – you know, like the
flashing neon signs in Times Square or Piccadilly Circus, not quite
Las Vegas standard, but flashing saying READ ME – was Isaiah
58:6—

> *"Is not this the kind of fasting I have chosen:*
> *to loose the chains of injustice*
> *and untie the cords of the yoke,*
> *to set the oppressed free*
> *and break every yoke?"*

Then I knew we were going to be in the right place and that I had
heard the Lord about the themes of 'Cry Freedom'. Verse 9 says,

> *Then you will call, and the LORD will answer;*
> *you will cry for help, and he will say: Here am I.*
> *"If you do away with the yoke of oppression,*
> *with the pointing finger and malicious talk...."*

In Houston I said, "We know that people who are here tonight
have been crying to the Lord, and he wants you to know that he has
heard you." First Dorothy read out the words that she had brought,
and then I read mine:

1. A lady with long blonde hair has come sceptically —hoping it
could be true that it is the Lord's will to heal, but doubting it very
much from her own experience.
2. A lady five feet three inches tall, with dark hair, has had a very
disturbing bereavement and does not believe the light will shine
again.
3. There are those who are very heavy in spirit. You are well read
and learned; you can teach the Scriptures and preach the gospel, but
have come to a place of not *knowing* his peace, not feeling —and,
looking back, it seems you have never felt the JOY that his presence
should bring. In his presence there is fullness of joy.
4. Someone has just been bested in a business deal and is feeling
very hard-hearted and vindictive. If you can lose that and ask for

forgiveness, then your peace of mind will be given back. It has made you very testy, very grumpy with your wife and family. Plus there is an even bigger deal in three months time, if you can release the malice.

5. A problem with the left elbow —it is seen as a white spot right in the middle.

6. A problem with the bowel – in fact the lower intestine – it is not cancer.

7. Osteoporosis – crumbling bones – you think it is inevitable as your mother had it.

8. The third vertebra —and the pain goes right through the shoulders.

9. Someone has been seeking, but doubting all that they hear, for a long time. They have a sort of irritation in the left side of the left eye. It sort of twitches in the eyelid. God is being specific because he wants to pierce through the doubts.

At that point I stopped reading and asked the man who had the twitching eye to stand up, because if he wanted to get rid of it and be certain that God had heard him and wanted to reassure him concerning all his doubts he could settle that there and then. The man stood up. His eye stopped twitching.

It was also confirmed clearly that we were so right not to have come earlier to be able to visit with members of the church. It transpired that the five foot three lady with dark hair was in the congregation with friends. Everyone in the place had recognised the word concerning her. The tragic bereavement that she had suffered had recently been in all the newspapers. God spoke to her through that word that night and she was able to start the journey towards the light. She knew that he had heard her crying. I was told later that she was able to be in court when the case was heard, and publicly stood and forgave the perpetrator.

Some of the comments of those present during the mission were sent to us from an article that was published in the church magazine. You will see the effect and worth of the prophetic ministry comes through clearly:

THE VICKERS MISSION

Each time there's a mission at our church we may ask ourselves, 'Is this for me?' Last weekend, September 10-12, the 'Cry Freedom' Seminar, led by The Reverend Randolph Vickers and his wife, Dorothy, was described on the brochure as 'A Weekend of Release'. For many of the 400 plus attendees who were set free from the emotional pain of hurt, fear, feelings of rejection, abandonment, and physical pain, the promise was kept.

At the beginning of the weekend, Randy and Dorothy spoke prophecies concerning members of the audience of whom they had no prior knowledge. These prophetic words were confirmed over the weekend as evidenced by the following testimonials of individuals who received healing, hope and freedom:

Sue Edmondson: "I could feel the weight and sadness lifted off my shoulders and heart physically... I now smiled and was happy. It was such a blessing and I will lean on it."

Katherine Edmonson: "It was a confirmation that good was present in my life."

At this powerful, spirit-filled mission, based on biblical teachings, Randy proclaimed, "Our freedom lies not in what we achieve, but only in the acceptance, love and significance that flows unconditionally from our Father God."

"Don't just take what we say as fact," they both cautioned during the weekend. "Check it out with Scripture yourself and tell us anything that is wrong. We solicit feedback, positive or negative."

Their message was received and manifested in body, mind and spirit. All of the gifts of the Spirit were present, bringing salvation to several, bestowing prayer language to those who asked, and offering the freedom that God promises to his children. But the most definitive words will be those of some of your fellow parishioners who were blessed to be there.

Lana Short: "Through the prayers offered by Reverend Vickers, I experienced an inner healing I had no idea I had need of. It was truly a freeing moment for me. The teaching was profound and I was blessed in many ways. It made me realize God has a mysterious way of providing for needs, known and unknown."

Terry Deckard: "The 'Cry Freedom' weekend with Randy and

Dorothy Vickers was like Christmas ... when I opened the present from my Daddy. It was exactly what I needed.

Bailey Family: "The Holy Spirit surrounded our family, uniting us in his healing grace. We were able to hear God's call, individually and as a family. As we forgave each other and ourselves, we received strength to build his kingdom by taking on forgiveness and letting go of fear...."

Raid Kirchen: "To have our resources constantly renewed is to be fully dependent on God for everything. Healing begins in community of acceptance."

Millie Wilson: "Lifetime of love rolled into one weekend...."

The Van Natta Family: "...my two daughters, Rachel and Rebekah, went for prayer Friday night and were filled with the Holy Spirit. This was the biggest blessing for Will and I to be part of. They are telling their friends without hesitation about the weekend. Two more for the kingdom of God."

Sandra Spencer: "What a powerful weekend. Blessings did abound. The Holy Spirit was so present – so there – for everybody. It was the best!"

Yvonne Heine: "I was gently lifted off my feet and especially blessed."

Leigh Bonner: "It was as personal as each person's faith...."

Other comments we received:

The Vickers spoke with quiet authority and ministered with amazing insight. Our weekend listening to them was very well spent and the course of our lives has been greatly altered by their visit.

I know God loves us and wants to be part of our lives, but I learned Friday night, he knows and cares about our thoughts and worries. God brought the Vickers to give me a personal word of comfort and reassurance. God knew exactly what I needed to hear at that moment and he spoke it: directly through Randy. What a blessing! What a gift.

I remember particularly one young married lady called Ellen who came for ministry on the Sunday evening in the sanctuary. Her husband was with her. As I spoke into her what the Lord was revealing to me, she was overwhelmed by his presence, and as she lay on the floor she was released —very, very loudly. She was only a little girl, but whenever she wrote to me after that she referred to herself as 'the little lassie with the big lungs', because even she was surprised at the volume of noise that came out. She later gave public testimony at an Alpha weekend. She said that she wanted to share everything that had happened on that night, having only given detail to her husband. She went into minute detail emphasising how, 'Randy had spoken of things that he had no way of knowing.'

Soon after arriving home, I received this in a letter from a lady. She wrote:

My husband Bill at my urging asked Randy for healing of his circulation in his legs and feet. The valves that control the flow of blood allowed the blood to "back up" causing severe varicose veins and discoloration of the feet. On Monday after you prayed, the right leg was 90% improved and the left, the worst affected one, was 60% improved. On Tuesday he called from work to say that in addition to his legs being so much better, a disfiguring, extremely bulging scar, which was the result of a car accident when he was 19, had flattened into perfect alignment with his leg and the raised red/purple incision was smooth and skin coloured! Praise God, a bonus!

We went to Houston again in 2003

We were invited to go back to Houston to lead a healing mission which was to take place in 2003. Dorothy and I asked the Lord whether he wanted us to go. Some months went by without either of us understanding that we had received any confirmation from the Lord. Then, in December 2002, as I was preparing for Christmas, I clearly knew that he wanted us to go to Houston as invited, and that the theme would be 'Released into Joy'. Now I knew what I had to teach at that mission, too: the great, central truths revealed in the Scriptures and confirmed in my own experience and that of countless believers. God chose us before the creation of the world (See Ephesians 1:4.) The original goodness of God's creation was marred by the terrible effects of the Fall, but there is a wonderful restoration available to everyone through Jesus, who is true God and true man: the light who gives light (see John 1); the radiance of God's glory. (See Hebrews 1.) Speaking of Jesus, at that time I said, *The celebration of his birthday is also the time of new beginnings, of new hopes. That is what his birthday means for us. So even if you do know my Jesus but have been feeling low – depressed – miserable – sick, with little hope for the New Year or in fact any year —this is the time to change tonight.*

The Lord showed me more that I was to say: *It is not just that we do not have to wait until Christmas to celebrate Jesus' birthday, but that this time of new beginnings is not like making resolutions for the New Year. It is not a 'refurbished second chance' thing. When ministering in inner healing I use a picture of a removal van with 'Renovations by God & Son' painted on the side, to illustrate that God is not in the business of knocking down but of renovation, but he showed me that this is only partially right. He is a builder of originals. He says that when we are born again we become a new creation.*

I spoke of the new creation that happens when we are born again by the Spirit of God, and of the true hope that is then ours —of a wonderful eternity shared with our God. And I contrasted the genuine joy of life in Christ with the desperate lack of joy I had seen in so many joyless lives today, in people who had tried other routes to fulfilment and discovered their emptiness.

I mentioned the struggles of some who had been in drug addiction, then offered this challenging, life-giving teaching for everyone: *Finally, brothers, whatever is true, whatever is noble, whatever is right, whatever is pure, whatever is lovely, whatever is admirable—if anything is excellent or praiseworthy—think about such things. Whatever you have learned or received or heard from me, or seen in me—put it into practice. And the God of peace will be with you* (Philippians 4:8f). *Set your minds on things above, not on earthly things* (Colossians 3:2).

At a ministry weekend for addicts, some time before, the Lord gave me a word for one young woman who was on heroin. I knew absolutely nothing about her. So at an opportune time (during a sharing of communion) I went over and told her that she did not need worry any more about her little girl, she was with the Lord and she was happy, so she need not mourn any longer. The woman burst into tears. "I have a little boy —I did not know I had a girl."

'Oops,' I thought, 'did I hear God wrongly?' But she went on to say, "It was all my fault. I had a baby and through my fault I lost it, I did not know until now that it was a little girl."

I said to her, "The Lord wants you to know that he has heard your sorrow and repentance and wants you to know that you are forgiven. Can you receive your forgiveness?" But in her misery and grief she could not. Strangely enough, that weekend I had been prompted to do something that I had never done before. I had blessed some water and taken it with me in a bottle, as well as the oil I often carry. I asked her what she would have called her little girl, and would she like to name her now?

"Oh, yes," she agreed. As she named her baby I poured the holy water on the woman's head. (It reminded me of 1 Corinthians 15:29, where we learn that some were baptised for the dead.) Then, as she asked for release from the vows she had made, I anointed her with oil. We then saw the prophecy in Isaiah 61:1–3 manifest in that room and in her. The Spirit of God was upon us. She, the afflicted, received the good news. She who had been captive in her grief was set free. She who mourned was comforted, and she received the oil of gladness instead. The mantle of praise was upon her. A beautiful smile wreathed her face and then the joy could not be suppressed. She started to laugh and she laughed without stopping for at least half an hour, and then at intervals throughout the rest of the day. The teaching continued—

That is what this weekend in Houston is about. This is what we are going to see in this place. You might think: 'But I am too weak, miserable, depressed to be joyful.' But the joy of the Lord is your strength, your fortress, your safe harbour.

We know that there is rejoicing in the presence of the angels of God over even one sinner who repents. (See Luke 15:10.) Each one of us is a sinner. Just think how much joy we can cause in heaven tonight when we come to repent. And then that joy, not your own manufactured, pitiful attempt at joy, but the joy of the Lord, will fill you. Yes, you are too weak now —but who lives in you? God lives in you. Rejoice in that, then he who has the strength, above all powers, will be your strength. This is not natural joy; this is not worldly strength.

We say, 'But I am too dry.' Even Isaiah, who did not have the joy of experiencing that new birth the way you did, says you can joyously draw water from the springs of salvation. (See Isaiah 12:3.) David wrote, in Psalm 51:12,

> *Restore to me the joy of your salvation*
> *and grant me a willing spirit, to sustain me.*

If you do not know that you are saved yet, then make sure about it tonight. Ask the Lord Jesus to come and be Lord in your heart right now.

The inheritance of joy is the birthright of the Christian. Who or what are you letting steal away your birthright, your inheritance? If you are in a tough spot, an awful situation, rejoice in hope; you have not yet seen the solution, but rejoice in hope. Be joyful in hope, patient in affliction, faithful in prayer.

Then I invited those present to join in a time of repentance, and we prayed, concluding with Romans 15:13,

May the God of hope fill you with all joy and peace as you trust in him, so that you may overflow with hope by the power of the Holy Spirit.

At the end of the Saturday morning session, I announced that we would have a time of prophetic ministry. Dorothy and I asked the Lord about the special things that he wanted to do.

I was given a word about a lady who had always wanted to die. After speaking this out I was called to the back of the hall to an elderly lady. The Lord showed me more about her emptiness and loneliness and unlovedness. As I spoke, the lady started to cry and so did her daughter who was with her. They told me that she had been diagnosed as having MS and depression, but I knew the cause went very, very deep. The Holy Spirit revealed that she had a broken heart and did not know how to love or how to receive love, even though she had a husband and children. Then she told me part of her story. She was a twin, but her twin brother had died in the womb some months before birth. Her parents, who had three daughters before her, had been longing for a boy. The boy was dead and they completely rejected this girl. In hospital the parents would have nothing to do with their daughter, so life continued for her in complete rejection. She told me that there was not one day in her life that she could remember waking up not sorry to be still alive —that there was not one day that she could remember not wanting to be dead.

I started to speak life into her broken and anaemic spirit. I cut her free from the wrong soul ties, spiritual ties and generational ties with her brother and her parents, committing her brother's spirit to the Father and into the blessed care of Jesus. I rebuked the spirit of death that had been with her from the time in the womb until the present, and told it to leave because she was choosing life. (See Romans 8:2 and Deuteronomy 30:19.) I asked Jesus to bring the time of her birth into the kingdom now, and into his presence and love where he could receive her and hold her safely and securely in a place where there was no rejection and fear. I asked the Father to give her a new heart instead of her broken and torn heart —a new big, juicy heart that could receive love without leaking. I asked Father to start filling her new heart with his love, and told her that this love was for her, just for her. As it overflowed, she could share it with others. I spoke into her spirit that God had prepared a big banqueting table of life for her, beside the still waters. (See Psalm 23.) I told her that the table was full of wonderful things just for her; that, as with the overflowing love, she could share it with others —but it was hers.

Her eyes started to shine. Her face relaxed and lost its deathly pallor. Her mouth started to soften. She released forgiveness to those who had hurt her, looked up at me and said that she wanted to choose Jesus and choose life —that, for the first time in her life, she wanted to live.

Her daughter cried tears of joy as she looked at and listened to her 'new' mother. She looked up at me and asked whether I knew her name. When I said that I did not she told me more of the story of her birth. In the hospital, as the parents would have absolutely no contact with her, the nurses needed something to call her, a name to write on the forms. Along with a bouquet of flowers was a card with the words 'Receive these with joy.' So the nurses had called her Joy, and that had remained her name throughout her life. Today we had truly seen life released into Joy. I had that wonderful sensation of knowing that I was right in the place, where God wanted me to be. We had truly witnessed the theme he had given me for the mission beforehand —'Released into Joy', which had been fulfilled before our eyes!

After lunch, Joy stood and gave her testimony. Over the days that followed, her friends told us of the dramatic change that they could see it had made in her life.

More of the prophetic touching lives

Prophetic ministry touches on so many aspects of lives, as well as the area of healing. Here is one illustration of that, from Sandra, who came to Beggars Roost. She later wrote this:

In 1998 I brought my mum to the Centre. She is not a Christian. She witnessed what Randy said at the beginning of the service: 'There is someone here facing a lawsuit. The Lord has said, 'Not to worry, it is settled.' I had prayer as I had a court case pending where I was pursuing personal injury compensation. The other side would not pay up, so my solicitor advised we go to court. Although the accident was not my fault, I was terrified at the prospect of appearing at court. About three weeks went by following the prophecy, and my solicitor rang me to say that he could not believe it, but the other side had come back with an offer. He was flabbergasted at how much they were willing to offer. I told him about God's word for me that it was settled and that he should accept what they offered. At this point my solicitor was still insisting and directing me to go to court. Again I told him that God has said that it is settled and that he should accept. I don't know what my solicitor said to the other side, but they came back with an offer for further costs of £470.00. Randy and Dorothy, I must report that the sum that God had arranged for me, without going to court, was in fact the same figure that my solicitor had said we should get if we went to court but with the additional £470.00.

7

TEACHING THE BASICS

Pumpkin Town 'revival' and 'Healing Mountain'

Pumpkin Town is the name of the community nearest to 'Healing Mountain', of which more below. Two years prior to our going to South Carolina, The Reverend Dr Pam Cole and her engineer husband Robbie Cole had given up precious time to come and listen to us talk in the Presbyterian Church in Laredo, and at YWAM headquarters in Tyler, Texas, on different occasions. They had been intrigued with our story of Beggars Roost and all that God had been doing there since we started in 1991. The vision the Lord had given us of going out and encouraging the body of Christ in his healing ministry really spoke to them, and they knew that this was work they were being called into. So they invited us to visit them and to inaugurate the healing ministry they felt that God wanted to plant there. In giving me permission to use part of their story, Pam emailed: 'What a joy to read your book! It is exciting to be a part of it. Your coming here was so important to us —and, as Robbie says again and again, our coming to Texas to meet you was a major turning point in our lives. I still believe that God intends to make Healing Mountain a sister to your ministry.'

Pam and Robbie bought around forty acres of a mountain to build their home and start their ministry. Robbie designed and virtually built the whole house himself. I mean it! He did not just assist the builders, he *was* the builder. The house that Robbie built on what I call Healing Mountain is so beautiful, on a wonderful tree-covered mountain. God was not only speaking to them, he was busy preparing a whole clutch of people to be part of a massive project.

Amy's vision

Amy is a nurse who loves horses and children. She had a vision to build an equestrian centre, where disadvantaged children and disabled children would be able to make friends with horses and learn to ride and be free for a while. Although Amy had been subject to a series of very unhappy events, we know it says in Romans 8:28, ...*in all things God works for the good of those who love him, who have been called according to his purpose.* This he did. Amy found herself with the backing to start to see her vision realised. She thought she had the place to build her dream, but it just was not working out. In the meantime Pam and Robbie had pledged all they had to buy some further acres of the mountain, to save the owner having to develop on it. When Amy's expected site was not working out, her attention was switched to the mountain. She was able to buy the acres Pam and Robbie did not need, and many more, from the owner, so that she had sufficient not only to build a huge stabling complex but also massive arenas, outdoor and covered. They looked bigger than those used for the riding competitions at the Olympics. The second floor holds a large meeting room where we held the teaching and ministry sessions, and the third floor was to be a large, attractive apartment for the manager. Amy will be able to develop trails for riding on the other land she has on the mountain, and will have no problem with her neighbours, Pam and Robbie, and other Christian friends who are now part of the healing vision. Mike and Ellen Johnson and Sue and Scott Edgar bought more of the mountain, and are planning to build houses among the trees. The Lord really is bringing a wonderful team together. He also provided a new husband for Amy, and Pam married them on the mountain in the week that we arrived. Gary Goudelocks (a paediatrician) and Amy are going to build a chapel on the spot where they married.

Pam had asked us to come over to South Carolina to help start the ministry in a barn. Then Sue wrote to warn us that the barn was not finished, was surrounded by red mud, and was still occupied by horses. So Dorothy and I were not quite sure what we were walking into. You can imagine our gasps of amazement when Robbie drove us over their beloved mountain in a four-wheel drive and we were met with the view of this magnificent building. We were thinking 'barns' as Englishmen think of barns: corrugated iron roofs on plank walls, with gaps between the boards to let the cold wind blow through. This, by contrast, was a splendid equestrian enterprise, complete with horses and hay rides.

Dorothy and I taught through the week on basic principles of Jesus' ministry of healing, and some of what follows in this chapter is based on those sessions. On the Tuesday, which was to become the infamous 11th September, remembered forever as the day of the terrorist attack on the USA, a whole group of us – including Dale and Mary Youngs with their children, and Cindy with hers, who had all come over from Laredo to be with us – had planned to go up to the town of Montreat, North Carolina. Montreat is famous as the home of Billy Graham, and houses a large Presbyterian college. That day, like many days which followed, was overshadowed by the events that took place in New York, Washington and Pennsylvania.

In the morning before we started to drive north to Montreat, we all met at Amy's house. We sat astonished and horrified as we watched the tragedy unfold in New York, as the aeroplanes crashed into the Twin Towers. Like so many, we could not believe what we were watching at first, somehow hoping this was a film animation, yet we knew in our hearts that this was actually happening as we sat there. Consternation and confusion reigned for a while, even in the calm security of a South Carolina kitchen. What could we do? What should we do? What was it right to do? The children were milling round in expectation of the outing that had been planned for the day, so we piled into the vehicles and set out for Montreat. Those of us without children actually in the car with us as we drove were able to keep our radios tuned to the news, and so heard the other details of the story as they emerged. It was so strange. It was rather like living in a parallel universe. Somehow it was as if we were each in two parts. One part of us drove through the beautiful, unspoiled countryside of the Carolinas, walked through the tranquil grounds of the Presbyterian seminary and tried to concentrate on everyday things, such as the best place to lunch to suit the kids, where to find toilets, and so on. Yet, simultaneously, the other part of us was acutely aware that, in states to the north, terror was wreaking havoc in the life of America.

In the evening, Dorothy's talk on knowing who we are in God

was most apt. We were able to pray and minister to many hurt souls and human spirits.

Because of the turmoil with the airlines it was decided that we should all drive back to Laredo on the Saturday. Pam negotiated the loan of the bus from the Presbyterian old people's home. This was a fifteen seater vehicle, used to transport residents to the town for shopping or local outings. It was certainly not designed to take seven adults and seven children fifteen hundred miles across four states in twenty-four hours. But with Robbie, Pam and Dale sharing the driving we travelled non-stop (except for food and bathroom stops) from Easley, South Carolina, to Laredo, Texas, starting at 9 a.m. on the Saturday from Amy's house and arriving at Dale's place about 10 a.m. on the Sunday morning.

Three basic essentials for a healing ministry

So you will understand how our first visit to South Carolina will live on in our memories. Our main aim on that visit was to provide a basis on which our friends could start and go on to build their ministry of Christ's healing on and around the mountain. Therefore, although we have prioritised 'Nine Basic Modules of Healing' for teaching at Beggars Roost, let me just outline three of them here, as we did in Pumpkin Town.

1. Knowing God's nature and his will to heal

Have you ever noticed what I think is probably one of the biggest healing events recorded in the Scriptures? I think that even if we had no further evidence than Exodus chapter 15 we could see that God's will for his people is that when they follow his word they will all be healed. The Hebrews had been treated as slaves for generations. A life in slavery was hard, and the Egyptians made the lives of the Jews bitter with hard work. We know from Exodus 12:37 and Numbers 11:21 that 600,000 men, as well as women and children, left Egypt on the night of the Passover. Various commentators suggest that this could mean somewhere between 1.5 million and 3 million people in total may have been involved. Had they enjoyed full modern medical care and a wholesome diet, in a population of that size we may well imagine that there there would have been many among them who were sick. I have no doubt that, in the hours before the angel of death passed over the houses with the blood of sacrifice painted on the door posts, there would have been some sick, fragile and lame. Yet, referring to the Hebrew people God brought out from Egypt, Psalm 105:37 tells us that among the tribes brought out by God there was nobody who was 'feeble'. This is made especially clear in the AV and NKJV translations of the Bible. (NIV has *no-one faltered.*) It would have been extremely surprising if, in that large population, there had been no frail people at all, no-one whose physical condition was such that they might have faltered, and in the natural we might think that would be impossible, but with God all things are possible. That the fact that none were 'feeble' is included in the scriptural account signals that something significant had happened. Then because of their disobedience when they did not obey God, all but three were to die during the forty years in the wilderness. Yet remember that it is also remarkable that, as we read in Deuteronomy 8:4, their clothes did not wear out and their feet did not swell during these forty years. I deduce that, at the great Exodus from Egypt, when God delivered his people from slavery, he healed all who were sick in that one night. And can you imagine all those old women walking through the hot desert for so long —and not even one swollen ankle, no sore feet and blistered feet? Does that not tell us something about a God whose nature and will is for his people to be well?

The biblical expression *Jehovah Rapha*, the Lord who heals, is of great significance here. *"If you listen carefully to the voice of the LORD your God and do what is right in his eyes, if you pay attention to his commands and keep all his decrees, I will not bring on you any of the diseases I brought on the Egyptians, for I am the LORD, who heals you"* (Exodus 15:26). The word *rapha* literally means 'to heal'. We are shown that it is God's very nature to heal as well as to bless. *Worship the LORD your God, and his blessing will be on your food and water. I will take away sickness from among you* (Exodus 23:25).

The Old Testament is full of God's promises to bless, heal and sustain those who follow and keep his word, e.g. Psalm 41:3, Deuteronomy 7:12–15 and so on. There is always the proviso that we have to follow and keep his word, because the truth is in the word. The life is in the word. (See Proverbs 4:20–22). Jesus told those who believed him that if they held to his teaching and really were his disciples they would know the truth and the truth would set them free. (See John 8:31f.) It is the word of truth, God's word, that sets us free, not our experience. The word tells us, *For nothing is impossible with God...* (Luke 1:37). Do I really believe that or do I just toy with the idea? Are you an *indweller* of the word, not only a reader and learner of the word? The Jews are sometimes referred to as people of the book. Their history is also our history as Christians, but for us it is much more than that, much greater than that. Scripture is complete and cannot be added to, but we are told of another book: the Lamb's book of life, and we want to be 'overcomers' and find our names in that book. We are church, we are the body of Christ, corporately and individually. We who are born again are the temple of the living God. We know that some end-time events which have been prophesied in Scripture, and to which the Book of Revelation testifies, are still to happen. Almost two millennia have passed since the closure of the canonical Scripture, but your life and mine are vitally significant in terms of what God is doing in his kingdom, and we need to be aware that the words of Scripture are just as much alive and active in our everyday lives now as they were when they were first written. Do remember that we look forward to our names being in that book which belongs to God alone. (See Philippians 4:3 and Revelation 3:5). Heaven is watching each of us: so always remember that your life matters very much to God.

We recall again that Isaiah prophesied what Jesus was coming to do for us (see Isaiah 61:1f); and how in Luke 4:1ff., following on from Jesus' baptism in water and the descent of the Holy Spirit upon him at that time, Jesus came out of the wilderness and returned to Galilee in the power of the Spirit. Then he entered the synagogue and applied that prophecy. Jesus was stating clearly who he was and what he had come to do. He revealed, too, that he only did and said what he saw the Father do and say. It was clearly being proclaimed and demonstrated that it was his intention and will to preach the gospel of the kingdom, and to heal the sick. It is the will of Father God that the gospel is preached and the sick are healed.

Having applied Isaiah's prophecy to himself, Jesus went on to prove he meant what he said. *Jesus left the synagogue and went to the home of Simon. Now Simon's mother-in-law was suffering from a high fever, and they asked Jesus to help her. So he bent over her and rebuked the fever, and it left her. She got up at once and began to wait on them.*

When the sun was setting, the people brought to Jesus all who had various kinds of sickness, and laying his hands on each one, he healed them (Luke 4:38–40). Jesus healed *all* who were brought to him. Matthew 8:17 teaches us that Jesus, in doing this, fulfilled the prophecy from Isaiah, that he *took up our infirmities and carried our diseases*. The Greek words for 'infirmities' and 'diseases' mean just that – there is a full physical dimension to the meaning – but undoubtedly, when Jesus is present, spiritual and emotional implications are also encountered.

What proof did he give John?

When John the Baptist was in prison, with his life in mortal danger, the question he had his disciples ask, *Are you the one who was to come...?* suggests that he started to wonder whether he had misunderstood something. Was Jesus really the Messiah? That can maybe help those who are still seeking, and who may assailed by doubts. John was born to be the forerunner of Jesus. His father was told that he would be filled with the Holy Spirit even from birth (Luke 1:15), and when his expectant mother, Elizabeth, was visited by Mary, now pregnant with the baby Jesus, John 'leaped for joy' in his mother's womb. So he 'knew' Jesus even before they were both born. Then his life was devoted to telling people about the Messiah who was to come. His whole life was centred around preparing people to meet with Jesus. John baptised Jesus in water and stood there in the Jordan and was witness to God speaking from heaven, declaring that Jesus was his Son, in whom he was well pleased. John knew in his spirit, had seen with his eyes, and heard with his ears who Jesus was. Yet even he came to a time of questioning. So he sent his disciples to ask Jesus was he really the one who was to come! Jesus does not get upset. Jesus does not give a long theoretical answer. Remember, in his talks to the people, how Jesus used the imagery of being able to tell what kind of tree it is by the type of fruit it bears. He is teaching that you can tell what the nature of a man really is by what he does. So he replies to John in the same vein. The fruit demonstrates the truth: *Jesus replied, "Go back and report to John what you hear and see: The blind receive sight, the lame walk, those who have leprosy are cured, the deaf hear, the dead are raised, and the good news is preached to the poor"* (Matthew 11:4f).

Often I get people saying that the salvation and healing on the cross is purely spiritual and emotional. They quote 1 Peter 2:24,

He himself bore our sins in his body on the tree, so that we might die to sins and live for righteousness; by his wounds you have been healed. The Greek word used for stripe means a wound that trickles with blood. The word used for 'healed' here means to cure, to heal, to make whole in the physical sense, as well as referring to salvation. We are talking 'wholeness' in every sense. That is why so many of my friends involved in this ministry refer to it as a 'wholeness ministry'.

Jesus demonstrated and stated his will, and had compassion

When asked by the leper if he was willing to heal, Jesus stated that he was willing. Jesus is the same now as he was then and will be forever. So, if it was his will then, it is his will now.

When he came down from the mountainside, large crowds followed him. A man with leprosy came and knelt before him and said, "Lord, if you are willing, you can make me clean."

Jesus reached out his hand and touched the man. "I am willing," he said. "Be clean!" Immediately he was cured of his leprosy. Then Jesus said to him, "See that you don't tell anyone. But go, show yourself to the priest and offer the gift Moses commanded, as a testimony to them."

When Jesus had entered Capernaum, a centurion came to him, asking for help. "Lord," he said, "my servant lies at home paralyzed and in terrible suffering."

Jesus said to him, "I will go and heal him" (Matthew 8:1).

Filled with compassion, Jesus reached out his hand and touched the man. "I am willing," he said. "Be clean!" (Mark 1:41).

Doctors and medication

I was talking with a Christian doctor friend (a general practitioner) about divine healing. He did not have a problem with the idea of Christian healing as such, but could not say that he believed that it was always God's will that people should be healed. So I posed a question that leads inexorably to a demonstration of the absurdity of that position, asking him how as a Christian he could continue to practise in a profession which led him continually into disobedience! The medical profession must operate on the assumption that healing or curing is good and is to be pursued. Does it make any kind of sense for Christians to hold that God sometimes wants people to remain unhealed? Scarcely, especially as we see throughout Scripture so much testimony to God's revealed will for healing. That doctor's way of thinking about God's will, had it been correct, would mean that in trying to help the patient he risks going against God's will in administering beneficial treatment! The same logic would apply to us all. If we do not think or feel that it is God's will that we get better, or if we think that God really gives us the illness or disability for some purpose (as some mistakenly suggest), then that would mean we should not seek to get better! On that erroneous premise we should not take any medication or do anything to alleviate the symptoms, as we would be going against God's will for us; we would be being disobedient, for, on that line of thinking, if it is not God's will that we should be healed then we should just get on and tolerate being sick and praise him for the sickness —not just praise him *in* our time of sickness but actually praise him *for* it. Needless to say, that would be a truly grotesque misunderstanding.

I hope very much you will agree with me that it is God's will to heal, so when we visit the doctor and take the medicine, and when we seek healing from God, we are acting in accordance with God's revealed will for us.

Are healings miracles?
I see healing as 'spiritually natural'; the body is designed by God to heal itself. Healing is simply restoring the body, spirit and soul to God's original design. I see a miracle as being some event which, on a given occasion, works in a way completely different to the normal or to our expectation.

2. Knowing our authority in Jesus
Accepting that it is God's nature and will to heal, we see from the following scriptures that it was his intention that Jesus would come into the world to make it possible for us to receive our healing through his death on the cross. In Isaiah 53:4–6 it was prophesied that on the cross Jesus would bear our griefs, our sorrows, our transgressions, our iniquities, and that by his wounds we would be healed. In 1 Peter 2:24 we get the confirmation that he bore our sins in his body, and that by his wounds we were healed. In John 10:10 Jesus states that the thief came to steal and kill and destroy whereas he came that we might have abundant life. This is confirmed in 1 John 3:8

where we are told that it is the devil who has been sinning from the beginning, and that Jesus came to destroy the work of the devil. And in Hebrews 2:14 we learn that Jesus shared in our humanity so that by his death he would *destroy him who holds the power of death*, that is the devil. It is recorded in John 19:28 that Jesus knew that all things had been accomplished in order that the Scripture might be fulfilled, and then he said, *"It is finished."* Then he bowed his head and gave up his spirit.

Following on from that, we need to be sure that we are able to continue in this work. He had first commissioned the twelve and then the seventy-two, giving them authority over unclean spirits, to cast them out, and to heal every kind of disease and every kind of sickness. (See Luke 9:1–6; Matthew 10:1–15; Luke 10:1–15.) Then in Mark 16:15ff, as we noted earlier, he taught that believers would lay hands on the sick, who would recover. We need to know that we follow in that line of authority and commissioning. So if we are to continue in his ministry of healing, we have to know that we truly are believers. It is not only a matter of believing in God and who Jesus is. We are told in James 2:19 that even the demons believe there is one God —and shudder. To me, it goes deeper than believing in Jesus as Lord, to a point that we need to be able to say, 'yes', if we are asked the question,'Do you believe Jesus?' —Not just believe *who Jesus is*; not just believe *in* Jesus but actually believe him and his word. In John 5:24 Jesus draws together the concept of believing his word and believing in God the Father. Do you believe that we can cast out demons, speak with new tongues, and lay hands on the sick (and they will recover)?

It would appear that to be in his ministry of healing I initially need to know two things about myself: that I am a believer, and that I am born again. *Jesus declared, "I tell you the truth, no one can see the kingdom of God unless he is born again"* (John 3:3). I need to know and claim for myself the promises that are involved in being a born again believer such as these:

1. That I have eternal life. (See John 5:24.)
2. That nothing can separate me from the love of God in Christ Jesus. (See Romans 8:38f.)
3. That he will do whatever I ask in Jesus' name. (See John 14:13.)
4. With *faith even as small as a mustard seed*, nothing will be impossible for me. (See Matthew 17:20.)

5. That I am a member of a holy priesthood. (See 1 Peter 2:5.)
6. That I am called as a saint. (Romans 1:7.)

I could go on and on reciting promise after promise of who the Scriptures say that I am in Christ Jesus, the promises that come with being a born again believer. I need to have the authority of who I am in Jesus written all through me, so that when it is necessary I can stand without fear or doubt against the wiles and deceit and force of the enemy. Then I know that Satan has to flee. (See James 4:7.)

One day, during a time of uncertainty in my life, God showed me a picture of a stick of candy rock. Usually these sticks of candy have the name of a holiday town written all the way through them in colour. Father told me to look at this stick of candy. I saw written through it, 'Randolph, son of God'. That is who and what you are, he told me. And no matter what happens to that stick of candy, whether it is snapped in half, sucked to the bottom, or broken into pieces, it will still say 'Randolph, son of God', right through the middle of it.

In this ministry we need that confidence as to our sonship and authority in Jesus, and this must be evident in the way we minister, for: *In this way, love is made complete among us so that we will have confidence on the day of judgement, because in this world we are like him* (1 John 4:17). So the love we show is to be like the love Jesus showed.

We need to know that we are Christians. Many years ago, a senior colleague was arguing with me about the fact that I had dismissed one of our managers. I had apologised for not informing him beforehand. He looked at me and said, "And you call yourself a Christian."

I was just about to let that go when I stopped and replied, "I don't call myself a Christian, I am a Christian. I might not always act like a good one but nothing can take away the fact that I am one." Having established that I am a believer, I have to know what the central work of a believer is. What do I have to do? Jesus said, *"The work of God is this: to believe in the one he has sent"* (John 6:29). That is so simple. Nothing complicated. Our job is to believe in Jesus, and everything else will flow out from that.

We noted that it was after the descent of the Holy Spirit that healings and miracles of Jesus are recorded. We also saw that he told the disciples to stay in Jerusalem until they received the same Holy

Spirit. The activity of the Holy Spirit is referred to in the Scriptures in a number of ways:

1. Promise of the Father. (Luke 24:49; Acts 1:4; Acts 2:33).
2. Gift of the Spirit. (Acts 2:38).
3. Baptised in the Spirit. (John 1:33; Acts 1:5; Acts 11:16).
4. Receiving the Holy Spirit. (Acts 8:17; Acts 10:47; Acts 19:2).
5. Filled with the Spirit. (Acts 2:4; Acts 9:17).
6. Coming upon. (Luke 1:35).
7. Clothed with power. (Luke 24:49).
8. Falling upon. (Acts 10:44; Acts 11:15).
9. Poured out. (Acts 2:33; Acts 10:45).

We have seen that the anointing breaks the yoke of oppression. We know that Jesus came to heal the sick, and that he did so. We know that Jesus has authority over everything. He said, *"All authority in heaven and on earth has been given to me"* (Matthew 28:18). The authority he gave to his followers in the commissions is the same authority he has given to us. He entrusted power to them to minister healing, and he entrusts it to us too.

It is Jesus' will that we are healed. Jesus came to destroy the works of the devil and when we minister in his name, in his love, we are doing as he did. We have noted already that according to John 14:12 the disciples were to do *even greater things* (than the *miracles* or *works* he did in his earthly ministry, depending on which translation is used). So in his name, operating in his love, the authority, power and will to heal is ours, and when we encounter the results of the activity of the devil, we enter that spiritual warfare covered by the victory Jesus won on the cross. He defeated Satan.

3. Be clear for prayer

If we are going to minister in the name of Jesus, and if we are going to pray and intercede for people, then we need to be sure that we are clear for prayer. Effective prayer needs: a Christian; the word; the backing of the power of the Holy Spirit. Before we start to pray we need to know that we are praying God the Father's will, and therefore can expect to receive the manifestation and fulfilment of our petition. When praying in relation to healing we should not add the rider 'if it is your will'. Using such a phrase is not showing humility. Not using such a phrase is not being presumptuous, because God's will in the matter has already been revealed. In the ministry of healing it is essential we understand that it is the nature and will of God to heal.

I have not found one passage in the New Testament where Jesus or a disciple *prays for* healing. There are numerous passages where they pray to God the Father before they minister in healing, but none where they *pray for* the healing. This is not splitting hairs. Prayer is to and with Father God. When asked how they should pray, Jesus told them in Matthew 6:9, *"This, then, is how you should pray:*
"'Our Father in heaven, hallowed be your name.....'"

In Psalm 139:23 we read: *Search me, O God, and know my heart; test me and know my anxious thoughts.* How many of us can stand before we pray and ensure that we have no anxious thoughts? How often Jesus tells us not be anxious. Just do not do it! He does not even suggest that we ask Father to take it away. It is something we have to do for ourselves because, as he says, *Who of you by worrying can add a single hour to his life?* (Luke 12:25); and, as Paul writes, *Do not be anxious about anything, but in everything, by prayer and petition, with thanksgiving, present your requests to God* (Philippians 4:6).

I could quote verse after verse saying virtually the same thing. Before you petition, stop being anxious. Fear and anxiety reveal the huge areas within our souls where we do not trust God. If we really, fully trusted that God would take care of everything and make it work for our benefit, then we would never again succumb to even the slightest twinge of anxiety. We get some clue of how to do this in this petition: *Create in me a pure heart, O God, and renew a steadfast spirit within me* (Psalm 51:10); and the resolution: *But in your hearts set apart Christ as Lord. Always be prepared to give an answer to everyone who asks you to give the reason for the hope that you have. But do this with gentleness and respect* (1 Peter 3:15).

Mercifully, we have a Father who is full of grace and mercy, and a Lord Jesus who was even willing to die for us to help us and do for us what we could never do in our own strength. This could be a very good time to ask Father to show you those things that you fear, and to help you get those fears out of your life for good. We have seen people healed of all kinds of fears, including: water, heights, men, flying, poverty, spiders and fire. We have seen release from agoraphobia, claustrophobia, and compulsive addictions such as going round time and time again, to make sure the doors are locked or that the fire is out, and so on.

When we respond to what God requires of us, then we can appropriate what he desires for us. We need to understand the foundational principles, centring on the two areas: **forgiveness** and **acceptance**, which are introduced here, and then we shall look at some practical examples.

Forgiveness

1. As we know, our own sins need to be forgiven by God. This forgiveness is so freely available to all who come to the cross in repentance, with faith in the saving blood of Jesus.

2. We must forgive everyone else who has ever sinned against us or hurt or harmed us. This is an unconditional requirement.

3. We need to appropriate personally, inwardly, the reality, the truth of what Christ has done for us in his finished work on the cross. Sometimes this is expressed as 'forgiving ourselves', but in truth forgiveness could only have been won for us by Jesus, and we know forgiveness when we bring sin to the foot of the cross. What needs to happen is to really accept at the deepest level of our being that we are truly forgiven people, so eliminating false shame and false guilt. We need to come to a place of assurance that the forgiveness described in (1) above is done, it is real, it is finished and complete, not retaining in our heart any residual guilt in relation to what has been forgiven by God. We are to accept the release which has been won for us, to truly enjoy the liberty that is God's gift for us.

4. We need to be released from any way in which we have blamed God for the bad things that have happened and that others have done to us. We may have asked why he did not stop the bad things happening. But we need to know that those bad things and bad actions did not come from God. They came from the disobedience of mankind, others' wrong choices, or from the enemy of God. God himself never hurts or harms us; he loves us with a perfect love. Sometimes what we have to do is expressed as 'forgiving God', but of course God does not need forgiving for anything. He is perfect, absolutely just, holy and merciful. We need to change our mind if our thinking has been wrong in this area; we need to be set free from the results of the blame we have wrongly ascribed to God; false declarations may need to be revoked, and countered with

postive affirmations of trust in him who is perfectly good and loving towards us, and always has been, even when we were totally unaware of his love and felt very trapped and hurt.

Acceptance

It follows from the points above that acceptance must operate in our lives in these ways:

1. We must accept God as he really is. See (4) above. Our minds are to be renewed as we study his word under the guidance of the Holy Spirit. Supremely, we begin to learn about the true character of God not from our own bad past experiences, which reveal man's sinful ways and this disobedient world, but rather from the truth the Father has revealed about his nature, in the person of Jesus Christ.

2. We must come to a real assurance that we are accepted by God. We may think ourselves unacceptable. If we had still been living in our sins, we would have been. But the Holy Spirit has led us to the point where we repented. God loved us so much that he has accepted us, and he is changing us, and he will go on changing us. Because we are *forgiven* sinners, we are acceptable to him; and not merely acceptable, but truly, lovingly, fully accepted as adopted precious children, members of his family. The hard thing is to change our minds and get used to thinking like this all the time! Compassionate ministry that constantly recalls us to the word of God on this point, and sometimes the deep work of the Holy Spirit, may be needed, to help us make this transition.

3. Flowing from this, we need to accept ourselves. Many are plagued and tormented by self-hatred, low self-image, low self-esteem, a sense of worthlessness. We need self-acceptance based on the sure foundation stated above.

4. We need to accept others. It is not enough just to have forgiven others. Our attitude to them must be like that of Christ Jesus. This can entail huge changes in all sorts of areas of our thinking, speaking and behaving. Acceptance does not mean approbation of all that others do; it does not mean agreeing with all they say. We are to be discerning and wise in our interactions with others. It does mean letting all our relationships be infused with godly, compassionate motivation. It does mean seeing and treating everyone else as having been created by God and loved by him, and sensing how he longs for them to come to know him as you have begun to know him.

Let us look a little more closely at what flows from some of those foundational principles.

We need to look at what is laid up in our hearts and overflows out to others. *The acts of the sinful nature are obvious: sexual immorality, impurity and debauchery; idolatry and witchcraft; hatred, discord, jealousy, fits of rage, selfish ambition, dissensions, factions and envy; drunkenness, orgies, and the like. I warn you, as I did before, that those who live like this will not inherit the kingdom of God.* (Galatians 5:19ff). That is how Paul describes what human beings are naturally like inside, and when we add this to all the hurt, abuse, resentment, loneliness, and so many other experiences that may have been ours along the way, it makes us very careful how we present ourselves to the world. So much of the anger, the hurt, the rejection, the loneliness and everything else that is there inside us, often well hidden and camouflaged, will have come through situations and issues involving others. With the help of the Holy Spirit we need to be able to look at this in the light of Mark 11:24ff. *"Therefore I tell you, whatever you ask for in prayer, believe that you have received it, and it will be yours. And when you stand praying, if you hold anything against anyone, forgive him, so that your Father in heaven may forgive you your sins. But if you do not forgive, neither will your Father who is in heaven forgive your sins."*

We need to examine all that forgiveness and unforgiveness means. In chapter 8 we address the matter of release from vows, particularly in relation to the breakdown of marriage. Such an important part of this release involves being able to forgive the other partner. When we do so we need to be aware of all that forgiveness entails. Take, for instance, a man leaving his wife for another woman after maybe twenty-five years of marriage. They have grown-up children. To the jilted partner what has happened often seems worse than a bereavement. It was a matter of will on her husband's part to leave. This is total rejection of her and all they have had together. It trivialises the past, the early years of courtship, all the words of love he has said to her, the joy of the birth of their children, the wonderment years as the children grew up, and the exchanging of gifts. So many memories have been trampled underfoot and sullied. The list is endless and the hurt is deep. Then there are all the practicalities of the present: dealing with lawyers, courts, settlements, money, where and how to live, what to live for. Again, the list can be endless. Then there is the matter of the future. But what future? What about all the things that they planned to do together when the children left home, when they retired; the joy of planning together for their daughter's wedding and watching him lead their daughter down the aisle. So many more dreams now trampled underfoot and sullied. There is so much to be forgiven. When I was thinking about all that can be involved in forgiveness amid such devastation, I had the picture of the old-fashioned cartoon character of a burglar: a burly fellow, complete with striped jersey, mask over his eyes and a large sack over his shoulder, labelled 'swag'. The caption to the picture was: 'Stolen from me'. That expresses the feeling perfectly. It can feel as though someone has broken into all that we held dear and ransacked the whole place; we feel vandalised, and we feel empty inside, bereft of all that was meaningful.

So forgiveness is to be able to acknowledge all of this, recognise its deep importance and then let it go —completely. Again, do remember in this sort of practical context that forgiveness does not mean condoning or agreeing with the actions of any who hurt or abused us. Forgiveness is not releasing them from their own responsibility before God for their actions; they will still have to work those things out with Father themselves, and seek forgiveness for their own sin against God's law. What we are forgiving when we forgive them is what we can forgive: namely the harm done to us. To do this has the effect of releasing oneself.

The other option, unforgiveness, is allowing the abuser to have control over your life. It is like locking oneself up in solitary confinement in a high security prison cell and handing them the key. Forgiveness enables us to take the key back, and with it control over our own future. Unforgiveness can take some strange twists and turns but keeps us from wholeness and joy. We saw this on another of our overseas visits. But first, a cautionary note:

A word of warning

It is extremely important to be aware that if there is talk of forgiving someone who is now deceased, this must not entail speaking to or attempting to communicate with the one who has died. That is absolutely forbidden in the word of God. What is meant by such an expression, in any case where the person concerned has died, is by an act of will, a personal decision, doing away in our *own* hearts with any resentment, bitterness or sense of a debt to be paid, revoking any negative words and confessions we have made about the person, and replacing those with beliefs, declarations, attitudes that are in line with God's word rather than our own often very hurt and damaged feelings.

So if we speak of 'forgiving' a dead person we are absolutely not to have some 'transaction' or 'communication' that involves them: we leave dealing with them to God alone, as has already been explained; we are to address what is going on in *us*, and we need to release ourselves from an ungodly heart attitude.

We went to The Hague: 'Honour your father and your mother'

Dorothy and I went to a European Convention of the FGBMFI. There came a time for ministry in the main convention hall itself and a man came over to me who was both very tall and quite large of girth. He said to me that he was born again and baptised in the Spirit but he did not know the fullness of joy. I laid my hand on his chest. Even if I had wanted to I could not have laid my hand on his head, as he was much too tall. I prayed to Father for enlightenment. I had to say to the man that he had to give his father the place of honour in his heart, as we are instructed to in the commandments. The man started to cry. "How can I do that?" he said. "I am Jewish, I am French, and my father was a collaborator in the war. How can I honour my father?" I replied something along the following lines: Because God says we need to honour our father and our mother, it is not optional. It is a commandment, therefore it must be possible. It does not mean that you condone or forget what your father did, you just honour him in your own heart. Without him you would not be you. God honoured your father with the precious gift that is you. Perhaps he did not know how to properly cherish that gift. But the Frenchman could still not do it. I then asked him whether he was he willing to be made willing. He agreed to this and so, rather along the lines of 'Lord I believe, help my unbelief', he prayed, "Lord I do not know how to honour my father, but I am willing to be made willing." There was a pause as I stood there with my hand on his chest. Then I felt rather than heard a rumbling starting in his tummy. This rumble developed more strongly and it coursed upwards through his large frame, finally erupting from his mouth in the loudest guffaw I have heard. He laughed and he laughed, as he now knew that fullness of joy!

Forgiving our son

Dorothy was away one Saturday and I was at home on my own. She had been given a pulpit from a decommissioned Methodist church, so I thought I would please her by re-erecting it in our Garden Room. Engaged in this, I was kneeling down when my back seized up. I was in excruciating pain. Only someone who has suffered on occasions with such a back problem will really understand how I felt. It was impossible for me to straighten up. It was totally impossible for me to even try to stand. I thought to myself that if I could crawl to the bathroom and lie in a hot tub for some time then it could possibly ease off. One big problem was that the bathroom was two floors above me. This meant that I had to mount two flights of stairs. I crawled to the bottom of the first flight.

Then I felt God reminding me of the anger still within me following a strong altercation at work on the previous day with my eldest son. Father showed me that I was still retaining strong resentment towards my son, and that I must forgive him and let the anger and resentment go. I readily prayed and asked Father's forgiveness, releasing complete forgiveness. Immediately, the crippling pain was lifted and I was able to complete the building of the pulpit.

Forgiving work colleagues

Dorothy and I went to speak at a meeting in a city some distance away. A man came forward for ministry. He said that he worked in an office but now his right arm had tightened up in pain so he had difficulty in writing. I prayed to Father and was then able to say to the man that he had to forgive. The man thought for a while and could not think of anyone against whom he held any resentment. So I asked the Holy Spirit to lead us further. I was then able to tell the man that he needed to forgive his colleague at work. "Well," the man blustered, "it is all his fault. He sits straight opposite me at work. He says he is a Christian and yet he sits and smokes and blows smoke straight into my face." After this tirade subsided he was willing to pray a prayer of repentance and forgiveness. We did not have to speak to his arm: it was healed as he forgave!

Some other kinds of forgiveness we may need to release in our hearts are described elsewhere, including forgiveness of churches and those in authority. The ways in which we will need to release are manifold, and no list can be exhaustive. The important thing is always to be ready to forgive. 'Seventy times seven' means always and everywhere. Forgiveness must be a way of life, because God has forgiven us and he requires us to forgive others freely, willingly, joyfully and instantly. He will give anyone grace to do it if they are willing.

We need to examine ourselves and ask whether we have left any opening for Satan or sickness to come in. Remember that Satan is the accuser. He is going to lie, steal, cheat, and do anything he can to destroy all that should be ours in Christ Jesus. We should not carry guilt, shame or condemnation.

We must be sure to have stored up in our hearts these precious truths: *Therefore, there is now no condemnation for those who are in Christ Jesus* (Romans 8:1). Why not? ...*because through Christ Jesus the law of the Spirit of life set me free from the law of sin and death* (Romans 8:2). And 1 John 3:21, *Dear friends, if our hearts do not condemn us, we have confidence before God and receive from him anything we ask, because we obey his commands and do what pleases him.*

I explained how I nearly put self condemnation on myself when accused by a colleague —I called myself a Christian and was going to carry guilt for terminating the employment of a manager. I have also told the story of the young mother who was in deep depression carrying guilt over the death of her daughter. We also need to be clear that we are not maintaining self-justification. So many of us try to cover our own sins by blaming someone else, or maybe the situation in which we find ourselves. Here are a few examples:

'I would go to church on Sunday mornings but all the family lie in bed late, so they prevent me from doing so.'

'If only my husband would become a Christian, then I could do Bible study.'

'If only my wife were more affectionate towards me I would not need to have an affair with the girl in the office.'

'If only my husband did not drink so much I could cut down as well.'

'If only everyone was nicer to me I would not need to tell lies.'

'If only I got paid more I would not have to cheat on the benefits.'

Just ask the Lord what your own 'if only's are. Then deal with the matter by repenting of the heart attitude, revoking the 'if only' and making positive faith-filled confessions instead.

Check out whether you or any of the family you know about has had any occult or secret society involvement. If so, go before the Lord, cut off and renounce any such links, and revoke any ungodly vows, pleading the blood of Jesus. Then ask for a fresh infilling of the Holy Spirit.

Have a check around the house to see if there are any artefacts, books, things that should not be there because of their connections and, if possible, burn them but in any event permanently destroy them. (Needless to say, you should not pass them on to anyone else!)

In Houston

On a Saturday morning I had done a session on blessings and curses and mentioned secret societies. Annie had prophesied about some freemasonry artefacts that some people had, including a box. That afternoon a brother and sister came forward to testify that they had gone home at lunchtime and destroyed a box which had held masonic regalia from a relative. Also, they were getting rid of a large portrait of a dead relative on which he prominently displayed his masonic ring.

At home

Literally in our own home, on the hearth, were two carved fertility figures which I had purchased when we lived in West Africa. Dorothy never liked these, and when we turned to Christ she was never happy with them in the house. As we learned more about the dangers of the occult, she became the more eager to get them out of the house but as they were mine she could not touch them until I agreed. When I said that she could dispose of them she took them into the garden and tried to chop them into pieces, but nearly wrenched her arm and could make no impression on them. Then she recalled that the Lord had told her to burn them but, try as she might, she was not able to set light to them. The Lord showed her that they were under the power of Satan so she prayed to break Satan's power, the figures flared up like tinder and were destroyed.

Check out whether you feel that others are more worthy or more needy, or have a better case to be healed than you. So many really nice people are ready to pray for others but feel that what they have is trivial, compared with the needs of others, to bother God. Then there are cases where some people are annoyed that others seem to get healed when they do not, and they think God must not love them as much as he does the others. That serious error causes much unnecessary grief. Remember that God is impartial. (See Romans 2:11; Acts 10:34). When you pray, be assured God loves us equally; he wants you to receive the healing that Jesus won for you on the cross as much as he does everyone else. He wants all to be saved and to come to a knowledge of the truth. (See 1 Timothy 2:4). And remember that he so loved the world that he gave his one and only Son, that whoever believes in him shall not perish but have eternal life. (See John 3:16). Believe that it is God's nature and will to heal.

As we taught on the basics of healing during the week of 9/11 in South Carolina, people were healed. A lady was set free from hay fever; T's leg was healed; F's back was released so that she could bend without pain; a lady was released from a spirit of oppression and Crohn's disease; Ellen was released from constant back pain; a lady's pelvic problems were sorted out. And more....

Following our second visit to South Carolina, in 2004, reports were sent to us after we returned home: A little girl had a bowel problem and was quite distressed as it hurt to go to the toilet. Following the prayer from the team in the barn, she is now having no problems and goes regularly and cheerfully. A young boy had suffered with nightmares and the team prayed with him. He had no more nightmares. A lady came with severe back pain due to an accident in a large supermarket. She also had diabetes, her eyesight was failing, and she had depression. After speaking into the trauma in her spirit, the Holy Spirit took over and rested her on the floor —and came in wave after wave upon her. When she eventually stood up, her eyes were shining; she said the warmth had come up from the soles of her feet right into her back, and it was healed. I have heard since we got back home that she says she still feels great, the depression has completely gone and her back is fine.

8

BABIES, MARRIAGE
AND VOWS

*Over the years we have had the pleasure of counting many babies as
Healing Centre babies. We have ministered to couples, or wives on
their own, who deeply desired to have their own children but who,
for a wide variety of reasons, had found it impossible. They have
either come to the Centre or we have met them when away from
home on ministry trips. Their stories show that although there can
be many reasons why people have not been able to conceive, nothing
is impossible with God.*

Jackie came to the Thursday healing service at the Centre one April
evening, at a time when she was feeling very low. She and her husband
suffered from infertility problems. She had given birth to a son with
medical help, but she and her husband had been praying for some
time that God would enable them to conceive naturally. There were
also other pressures on their marriage, which were damaging their
relationship. She wrote to us a couple of months after her visit, to
thank us for the prayer ministry she had received, and to say that the
marriage relationship problems had now been solved and that she
was much happier.

Jackie had been struck on that Thursday night by part of the
teaching which had dealt with the difference between being 'in
faith' and being 'in hope'. As she prayed over the following days,
she realised that she had not been completely 'in faith' that God
would enable her to conceive naturally. So she started praying in

accordance with Mark 9:24, *Immediately the boy's father exclaimed, "I do believe; help me overcome my unbelief!"* When Jackie had been at the Centre she had told us that she had been dwelling on Hebrews 11:11. This verse tells how Sarah had conceived through faith, even though she was well past childbearing age. Dorothy had told Jackie that Abraham had a promise from God which enabled him to have faith. The relevance of this to her situation was confirmed for her with Psalm 113:9, *He settles the barren woman in her home as a happy mother of children. Praise the LORD.*

Finding other Scripture verses – 'do not fret' and 'trust the Lord' – Jackie committed the whole thing to God, left it to him and stopped fretting about it. He was most gracious and took her to Psalm 128:3, *Your wife will be like a fruitful vine within your house; your sons will be like olive shoots round your table.*

In June, Jackie discovered that she was pregnant. Despite a number of complications, including a threatened miscarriage, she kept reminding herself of the promise. Her daughter, Rachel, was born, and later she and her husband went on to have another natural conception, resulting in the birth of their second son, Samuel. Through it all, Jackie began to realise how much she was loved by God. Like so many people, she had not felt that she was sufficiently important to God for him to listen to her and speak to her. She is certainly listening to his voice nowadays.

John and Mary came to Beggars Roost
This is their story as Mary told it.

John and I were married in 1993. We discovered after a couple of years that we were having difficulty in conceiving, and approached our GP, who was happy to refer us and to have a range of tests performed. We discovered that there was no medical reason for the infertility problems which we were having, which was reassuring, but this also meant that there was no treatment which we could undertake to help us in our situation.

1996 was an eventful year for us. It seemed that everywhere we went, God was speaking to us. We attended a Vineyard Conference in St Michael-le-Belfry in York, the New Wine conference in Somerset, and also attended an Ellel Ministries weekend for childless couples, at Glyndley Manor. On two occasions, the same passage in the Bible was read: Isaiah 54. Each time, the speaker felt that it was important to pray for couples who were unable to have children. We found these experiences very helpful, but the infertility problems remained.

In December 1996, we started visiting Beggars Roost in Stocksfield. I was having a great deal of trouble with upper back pain and was on sick leave from work at that time. Then, unexpectedly, I became pregnant in January 1997. We were elated, and immediately started making plans for this much longed-for baby. Sadly, I miscarried very soon afterwards. We found this experience of grief very difficult to come to terms with. A few weeks later, we visited Beggars Roost again. During the meeting, someone had a word of knowledge about miscarriage. We knew that God was speaking to us, and we were able to receive prayer about our loss and about our longing to have children.

During the next few weeks, God led us through an intensive time of prayer together as a couple, and showed us many areas to pray about. About two months after the miscarriage, I discovered that I was pregnant again. This time the pregnancy proceeded without difficulty, and I gave birth to a healthy baby boy in December 1997.

God used many people and many different situations to work in our lives especially during the year before our son, Jonathan, was conceived. We are grateful to everyone who took time to pray for us, and are so thankful to God for the ways in which he led us in prayer during that time. Every baby is a miracle, and we feel especially aware of that.

We went to Houston

In a previous chapter I mentioned Ellen, who attended the Cry Freedom weekend. She wrote us this encouraging letter.

Hello Dorothy and Randy,

...I had stopped infertility treatments after five long (gruelling) years of trying. We had joyfully started adoption proceedings in March, when SUDDENLY I discovered I'm pregnant.

God has given us a miracle, and I'm 15 weeks pregnant. The baby is healthy, and the heartbeat is strong. I was experiencing morning sickness and nausea (HOORAY for a healthy pregnancy!), but I'm feeling better and better every day.... It's been an amazing journey since the Cry Freedom weekend healing, and God has so graciously healed many, many emotional and spiritual wounds before he healed me physically. My marriage is intimately stronger, and we've felt God's tender presence so strongly in the last five years. In addition to infertility, we've had many, many trials, lost both of Stephen's parents within a year, had our house flooded twice, etc., etc. Throughout all the trials, God has increased our faith, and we've learned that he is trustworthy....

Finally, on a funny note, obviously God has worked on me quite a bit on the issue of control after my battling infertility. While in treatment, I never did a treatment cycle in February or March because I always thought it would be too hectic to have a baby in December with all the holiday preparations and hoopla ...the baby is due December 17th. Stephen fully expects the baby to be born on December 24 or 25th! ...we've certainly changed our minds and think having a baby this year will be the best Christmas present ever (aside from God's Christmas baby 2000 years ago!) Looking forward to seeing you in September and having you pray over the baby in my much bigger (by then) belly. Our Father had the perfect plan and timing all along! God is good, and the One who promised is faithful! Warmly, Ellen Tuffly (the little lassie with the big lungs!)

Fiona came to Beggars Roost.

Fiona came to the healing service one Thursday evening. She was in severe pain from an arthritic problem. Fiona longed to have a baby but the medication that she needed to take to control the pain of the arthritis was so powerful that it would cause great complications for any child that she might conceive. Therefore she was longing to be set free from pain. On the first occasion that she came there was certainly no evidence of any healing. For some reason I was led to ask her to return the following week but to come and speak with me before the meeting started. I still do not know why we needed to meet together before the meeting because again I had no insight into the root of the problem. During the normal ministry time that night, again there was not the slightest evidence of healing.

After the meeting was over and everyone else had gone home, Fiona was talking with Dorothy in the Garden Room. I joined them there because I just knew that we had to pray again. This time, as Dorothy and I prayed for guidance and I spoke to the problem, we literally, physically, heard her bones crunch, and could see and feel her bones moving into place within her, through her clothes. It was a phenomenal thing to see and hear. We heard from Fiona again the following April, when she wrote this.

Dear Randy and Dorothy,

As God has definitely worked in my life since my healing in September at your Centre, I felt I should write and let you know of the happenings. God has certainly shown me that when you put your trust and faith in his hands he does not let you down.

In January this year I made a firm decision to cease taking the remaining tablets I was taking for my back. Although initially I was unsure, I knew that if my strength resided in the Lord I would win through. And praise the Lord I gradually counted the days down into weeks and without any aches or pains! Eventually I reached a point where the doctor was happy for Tim and I to try for a family. In prayer also at this time I felt very much assured by God that this was his will and my desires would be given. This was further confirmed when a Christian friend shared with me that God wished her to point me at Psalm 37:4, 'Delight yourself in the LORD and he will give you the desires of your heart.'

Now my faith was deep rooted and I thanked God for the assurance. Needless to say I fell pregnant immediately! At present I am in the early stages of pregnancy, expecting a baby sometime around 1st December. However, this week I have had slight complications, which have unsettled me a bit, therefore I would be grateful for any prayer for the birth of a healthy baby and an uncomplicated remainder to my pregnancy.

I felt I must share this with you as it is thanks to the assistance at the Centre of prayer for Christian healing that I first began this journey that has brought me to this point, so thank you and may all the glory be the Lord's. Love in Christ, Fiona.

[A healthy baby was born in November, three weeks early.]

Kota Kinabalu, Sabah, Borneo

I went to work with The Very Reverend Koo Tuk Su, Dean of All Saints' Cathedral, Kota Kinabalu, Sabah, Malaysia for four weeks in 2001. Sabah is the country, which covers the northern coast of the island of Borneo. The Dean had organised a time of fasting, teaching and ministry for the period of Lent and invited me to be part of the team. As I am rather advanced in years, Dean Koo particularly requested that I spend most of my time working with the 'Golden Saints' (the wonderfully apt and gracious name that has been adopted by the senior citizens of the congregation).

Most of my teaching sessions were concerned with the gifts of the Spirit and the ministry of healing. In one particular period of around ten days we saw various healings, notably a number of back problems, and some were released in the gift of tongues; some thirty people were baptised in the Holy Spirit. Working with Dean Koo and all those Christians hungry for God was one of the most thrilling months of my life.

One lady who had come to one of the sessions on the work of the Holy Spirit was so enthused she encouraged her two daughters to come too. All three received baptism in the Holy Spirit and were eager for more. Elizabeth, one of the daughters, told me of the difficulty that she and her husband were having in conceiving a baby. They had been trying for over seven years.

I therefore arranged to teach some special sessions about generational sins, generational ties, soul ties and spiritual ties. There was a ministry time at each session and a number of people were set free from ancestral sin and all its possible involvement. We covered blessings and curses and people were set free. Another subject that we covered was that of vows, because people are so unaware of the danger and bondage into which they can place themselves even with some of the completely meaningless and foolish vows, promises and covenants they make. Marriage vows are of special significance. The couple promise that they will love, honour and cherish their partner until death. Divorce clearly means breaking this vow, but how about all the other segments of the promises involved — to love, comfort, honour, cherish, keep in sickness and in health, forsaking all others? Breaking any of these promises is breaking a vow and must be attended to accordingly. The Bible contains warnings in this matter of vow breaking. The breaking of vows can be a determining factor in childlessness. But God is gracious and merciful, and we can be released from our vows, as I will show in greater detail later.

I then held a separate session just for Elizabeth's family so that her husband would feel safe to attend. Together with her mother they were able to go through the details of her side of the family and cut themselves free from any ungodly associations. The husband was Chinese and the family on his side was Buddhist and was still involved with ancestral worship. He was able to cut himself free from all these associations. Together they were then able to receive blessing and promises of God, like those described in Deuteronomy 28, ...*All these blessings will come upon you and accompany you if you obey the LORD your God: You will be blessed in the city and blessed in the country. The fruit of your womb will be blessed....*

I returned to Sabah in June the following year, to be greeted by Erin, his proud parents and his grandmother. God gave the precious gift of life within weeks of their being set free from ties that can bind.

A new heart
When I went to Sabah on the first occasion one of the Golden Saints asked for prayer for a new heart because she had been diagnosed as having severe heart problems. When I returned in July 2002 she told me how, following the time of ministry, she had kept her dreaded appointment at the hospital during the week after I left. The doctors had given her an angiogram so that they could more clearly decide the procedures that they would follow. To their surprise, and her delight, this showed that her heart was perfectly well and fit, and there was no need for treatment or medication of any kind. When I met her that following year she was still praising God for her new heart.

They came to Beggars Roost
Matthew's parents first came when Mohini, his mother, was pregnant. They had heard that he was going to have club feet, and that there could be other problems related to his deformity. They brought Matthew to the centre when he was a very tiny baby, only a few weeks old. They told me that both feet were affected. Club foot is a congenital deformity in which the foot is twisted so that most of the weight rests on the heel. I must admit that I had to take his parents' word for it because to me a young baby's legs just dangle, and it is virtually impossible for someone who is not a paediatrician to diagnose.

One of the things that I have learned through experience is that, when confronted with congenital disorders, the place to start ministry is not with the baby, even if the person affected is now an adult, but with the parents. I think that you will find this holds good even when the person afflicted is in their 70s or 80s and their parents are long dead; you still have to start with what was happening pre-birth, prior to, during or after conception.

One of our team held Matthew whilst I talked with the parents. I asked them if there was anything that did not seem to be right that had happened whilst his mother was carrying the baby, or during the birth. Had they been alarmed about anything? Were there any traumatic shocks of any kind? Were they frightened about any situation? It transpired that, since they knew whilst he was in the womb that Matthew had club feet, the fear was whether there was anything else wrong, although a few of the major problems such spina bifida were ruled out by the time of delivery.

Mohini and her husband readily asked the Lord to forgive them for their fear. As they did this, Mohini says that Matthew's left foot did improve, and was considered best left until later; but it was not completely healed. It was almost a year to the day when I saw them again. The left foot had been partially healed the previous year; now they were due to go to the hospital during the following week for surgery on the right foot. Again I could not visibly tell whether anything happened that night, but Mohini telephoned the following week. She told me that when they went in for the operation the consultant told them that rather than operate he would send them home. He told them how to strap up Matthew's foot and instructed them to come in two months for a check up. Although Matthew did have strapping for a time, and could walk, his feet were not as good as they should have been. So about 20 months later he had surgery on both feet. In the event, God has used skilled surgeons to rectify the problem and Matthew's feet continue to draw admiration at the way they have been corrected.

Matthew's mother wrote, saying:

I think the main healing was for myself because when I first came to Beggars Roost I was afraid and partly angry and sad that my baby was going to be deformed. However I felt God's peace in my heart and knew all would be well —not necessarily that Matthew would be made whole. Right through Matthew's treatment I felt God's peace and reassurance, even when taking Matthew down to theatre. As a young boy Matthew has shown a great love for Jesus which only by God's grace is growing stronger. He is a very happy and loving child and shows concern for his mates and fellow human beings. Who

*knows what God's plans are for him. We can only pray and trust
that these will be revealed in time.*

Hindrances to conception.
In the case studies presented we have seen a number of the areas
that may need attention before conception can take place: stress in
relationships; stress in general; unbelief; lack of trust in God's word;
other medical problems; ungodly soul ties; generational sin; vows;
curses; fear; trauma.

As with all ministry, we must first ask Father to show us and lead
us, by the Holy Spirit, to any areas in the lives of the people that
possibly need to be healed before we reach the main petition. So
often in my experience, when these unforeseen areas are dealt with,
there is no need for further ministry. The matter is closed.

One more area which I have mentioned elsewhere can affect
conception, as well as being a hindrance to wholeness in general,
namely any connection that a person may have had with the occult. I
include involvement in these areas:
a) Such practices as reading horoscopes and fortune telling or
divination of any kind; seances; mediums; reading of tea leaves or
coffee grounds; crystal balls; ouija boards; tarot cards; connections
with or attendance at spiritualist meetings, etc.
b) Involvement with secret societies, including freemasonry and
associated organisations.
c) Involvement with elements of non Christian or pagan religions,
either directly or through such activities as yoga, various martial arts,
use of mantras and chanting.
d) Involvement with various so-called complementary medicines
and therapies or semi-medical practices such as homeopathy or
acupuncture. I am not saying that all complementary therapies are
of occult origin, but I suggest that anyone considering the use of any
such practices should carry out adequate research to clearly ascertain
their provenance.
e) Playing fantasy games. Once a mother telephoned me to ask
me to minister to her son who was about 14 years old. He had
been a smart, outgoing affectionate young chap but had now 'gone
very strange'. He was hearing voices, having nightmares, and had
withdrawn from the family. On the way round to their house I
picked up the pastor of their own church so that he could be fully

involved. When we got there we found that the boy was deeply involved with a fantasy game. He did not just play it himself. He had progressed to a senior position where he was the leader of a group of boys, and he actually invented and devised the situations and conditions of play. He was very frightened by what was happening, and as he was also a good Christian boy he realised something was not right and was ready to come to God in prayer and ask forgiveness for anything that he had done to offend him. We were then able to take authority over the evil that was oppressing him and command it to go and not to come back, as he had been forgiven and washed clean by the blood of Jesus. He was willing to close the door by agreeing not to play the game again. To his mother's joy, and his relief, he was immediately restored to his old self.

Other common factors can be: premarital sex; at some earlier age deciding— never to have children or never to get married; at an earlier age deciding that there was an inability to raise children; an early hatred of babies (perhaps following the birth of a younger sibling who seemed to usurp one's place in the family); abortion; miscarriage; delaying conception for career, or until a home could be afforded, or until one felt secure, or until one had travelled —and so on. Fear of conception or some of its ramifications (pain, sickness, loss of figure, loss of partner, lack of money and so on); sexual relationships forbidden in Scripture.

The vows we make

In my Bible I found 69 verses about vows, 118 verses about oaths and 55 verses about swearing, so clearly this is an area that we are meant to address. This subject really follows on from that of blessings and curses, which I have only briefly mentioned in this book when they have directly related to the stories being told. The two subjects are closely connected but, as was evident earlier in this chapter, it is imperative that we realise the impact that vows can have on our lives and health.

So much of this is about 'proclamation'. When we make statements we need to be acutely aware that somehow, somewhere, they will be tested. They boasted that the Titanic was unsinkable. Have you ever tried going on a diet and proclaiming that you are going to lose weight? When you start dieting you do not have to wait long for the testing. It comes thick and fast: food temptation such as you never thought possible! What is proclaimed has consequences.

Following our initial visits to the USA, one of the subjects that I realised I needed to look at more closely was that of vows and their relation to divorce. Although divorce may be as prevalent in the UK as it is in the USA, there are many more churchgoing, born again Christians in the USA who come forward for ministry. Central to marriage are the vows that we make, one to the other, in the sight of God. However, like most of God's laws, which were made for the good of society and our ultimate wellbeing, whether a person believes in God or not, we all need to obey his commandments —because whether you agree with his word or not, it is still his word, and is immutable.

Courtship is the time to test out whether or not we are compatible with one another. I do not include sexual activity as part of courtship. Sexual intimacy should come after marriage. As far as I know there is no statistical evidence to show that divorce is less frequent for marriages which follow after trial periods of cohabitation with one or more partners. As I write, the British government is seeking to enact legislation giving cohabitation legal standing similar to that of marriage. The government is going even further against God's strictures by recognising same-sex partnerships.

As to marriage vows previously made by divorced people, unless they are dealt with, the links are still there, and will affect every subsequent relationship. The scriptures exhort, *Above all, my brothers, do not swear—not by heaven or by earth or by anything else. Let your "Yes" be yes, and your "No," no, or you will be condemned* (James 5:12).

God means this —even if we mistakenly believe that oaths and promises not made in church or before a minister do not count. God is omniscient, so that, whatever we do or say, we do it in the sight of God. *If you make a vow to the LORD your God, do not be slow to pay it, for the LORD your God will certainly demand it of you and you will be guilty of sin.... Whatever your lips utter you must be sure to do, because you made your vow freely to the LORD your God with your own mouth* (Deuteronomy 23:1ff.)

Whatever we utter, we have to follow through —or repent and seek release from ungodly vows. God's law and commandment is relentless in its stand that marriage is for life. The healing of relationships is a priority. Civil proceedings may bring a marriage to an end, and the courts may declare that we are free to remarry —but in the sight of God the parties are still joined together; as we see when we look at soul ties, the couple is still 'one flesh' in the eyes of God. *"For this reason a man will leave his father and mother and be united to his wife, and the two will become one flesh.... So they are no longer two, but one. Therefore what God has joined together, let man not separate"* (Matthew 19:5f.)

When man and woman are united in the sexual act they become one flesh, even in the act of prostitution, where there was no intention by either side to become man and wife. They still become one flesh spiritually. Paul wrote, *Do you not know that he who unites himself with a prostitute is one with her in body? For it is said, 'The two will become one flesh'* (1 Corinthians 6:16).

The bond between a man and a woman continues after they have parted company —until God frees them following their repentance. Divorce breaks the bond, but does not render the vows void. Jesus' teaching was clear: *"It has been said, 'Anyone who divorces his wife must give her a certificate of divorce.' But I tell you that anyone who divorces his wife, except for marital unfaithfulness, causes her to become an adulteress, and anyone who marries the divorced woman commits adultery.*

"Again, you have heard that it was said to the people long ago, 'Do not break your oath, but keep the oaths you have made to the Lord.' But I tell you, Do not swear at all: either by heaven, for it is God's throne; or by the earth, for it is his footstool; or by Jerusalem, for it is the city of the Great King. And do not swear by your head, for you cannot make even one hair white or black. Simply let your 'Yes' be 'Yes,' and your 'No,' 'No'; anything beyond this comes from the evil one" (Matthew 5:31–37).

"Anyone who divorces his wife and marries another woman commits adultery, and the man who marries a divorced woman commits adultery" (Luke 16:18).

It would seem that if a single man marries a divorced woman, he commits adultery, because she is bound by vows to her first husband. If divorced for any other reason than the biblical one, she is still bound by her vows and is one flesh. Adultery may destroy the marriage bond but it does not abolish the vows. When a man commits adultery he is offending against three parties: the person he is with, his wife, and God. The same, of course, applies to an unfaithful wife. God wants to heal and restore relationships. That is his will, and therefore it is possible. For restoration, husband and wife need to be committed to doing God's will and obeying his principles, whatever it takes. Then he can heal estranged marriages. He invites us to bring him into all the problems which we cannot handle ourselves. I am going through all this because I do not want anyone to think that there is a quick and easy way out. As I say about curses and evil spirits, for a curse or demon to alight there has to be a landing pad within us in the first place, which has made us vulnerable and open to invasion. For forgiveness to be received and absolution given then there has to be true confession and repentance from the heart. I am not talking about remorse but repentance. So many of us look upon remorse as being the same thing as repentance. We go around looking miserable, governed by our feelings, saying we are sorry and that we wished we had never done it or never said it. Remorse stays in the mess, in the sin, in the bondage. Repentance, on the other hand, is an act; it is of the will, and it means making a decision. Repentance is acknowledging the sin and bringing it to the cross of Christ which alone avails for the sin, asking for and receiving his forgiveness, then leaving it behind and moving on in power and the grace of God, into his future for us.

I know that God can restore estranged marriages. He restored mine with Dorothy when I had done virtually everything possible to wreck it. Remember all authority and power is in Christ Jesus, and when we pray, in just the same way as when praying for healing we need to be sure that we are clear for prayer as is discussed in chapter 7.

Of course, Christians are not perfect and divorce is all too common amongst them. When they are divorced they face new challenges. God knows we need a spouse rather than go through life celibate but aflame with passion, as Paul acknowledges: *Now to the unmarried and the widows I say: It is good for them to stay unmarried, as I am. But if they cannot control themselves, they should marry, for it is better to marry than to burn with passion* (1 Corinthians 7:8f.) It was God's idea that a man should have a female partner, and he designed marriage in the first place. The Greek word *agamois* translated as 'unmarried' does not simply mean a single person but a person not in the state of wedlock, whether they have been previously married or not. Paul is not sanctioning changing one spouse for another, but his words offer some encouragement to those traumatised by divorce —to pick up the pieces of their lives and start again. It can be the extreme of rejection for a woman or a man to be divorced and left by their spouse against their will, and often with no idea that something was wrong. They may have no idea that their partner of many years had found someone else. This can be worse than had their partner died, because this is grief and mourning for a marriage that has been killed, and they have been rejected. The jilted party is confused, and wonders what was wrong with them, whether they were ugly, useless and incapable. They can feel that it must have been their fault; there can be self-condemnation and unforgiveness. Not only is there the past to mourn for but, as we have seen, all the future together that they are not now going to have.

We have not space here to deal with all the problems that arise for any innocent children from such separations. We knew two families where the partners split and each went to live with the spouse of the other. It was decided that the girls would go with the mothers and the boys with the fathers. Now is that not a sanitised way of arranging to split children from their own siblings? But the thinking got even crazier. One of the little girls became very upset because she was moving out with her mother but her dog was staying in her original home. So her mother explained to her that it would be too cruel to make the dog leave the home it knew just because she was moving. The emotional state of the dog was considered to be more important than that of the child. In this sort of situation we not only need to minister to the wounded soul but also to the wounded spirit which has been crushed. Their own very personhood has been abused and denigrated.

Then we minister to many caught up in all kinds of bondages such as pornography, self-mutilation, self-abuse and, particularly, self-condemnation. These are not necessarily caused through divorce but can have many starting points of which divorce can be one.

So how do we get ourselves out of this whole mess and get clear to marry again without taking the previous marriage into the future with us? Can it be possible? We need to look to the Scriptures for precedents. We find that David was forgiven for his adultery with Bathsheba, and in fact their second son became the great King Solomon, renowned throughout the world for his wisdom. Abraham was forgiven for his adultery with Hagar. Judah had a baby by his daughter-in-law. Rahab the prostitute was rehabilitated, and was part of the lineage of Jesus. In Revelation 2–3 and elsewhere in the New Testament we read of opportunities God gave to Christians to repent. This is his revealed character as we see in consistent biblical witness. God mercifully gave the pagan peoples of Canaan something like 500 years to get their act together before he sent in the Israelites. He gave the Israelites centuries to get their act together before the Diaspora. He gave Nineveh another opportunity after Jonah warned them. Is he going to be watching your every move? (He is!) But is he constantly punishing us for our offences, as some people think? If you think that, then you need to start to get to know him better. His will is always for the sinner to repent and be restored, and he provides opportunity for this. In Revelation 2:21, he says of Jezebel, *I have given her time to repent of her immorality, but she is unwilling....* He had given her an opportunity, but that opportunity always has to be accepted and acted upon for forgiveness and restoration to follow, otherwise there is indeed punishment for sin.

Marriage is God's picture of the relationship of Jesus with his church —Jesus' relationship with us, with me, with you; a very deep, intimate, individual relationship. Read Ephesians 5:22–32, which gives a very good foundation for what we need to know about marriage relationship.

We return now to the matter of vows. There are many verses in Scripture concerning vows, oaths and swearing. In Ecclesiastes 5:4, we have: *When you make a vow to God, do not delay in fulfilling it. He has no pleasure in fools; fulfil your vow.*

Jesus said, *"Again, you have heard that it was said to the people long ago, 'Do not break your oath, but keep the oaths you have made to the Lord'"* (Matthew 5:33). He also said this: *"But I tell you that men will have to give account on the day of judgment for every careless word they have spoken"* (Matthew 12:36).

The making of vows, promises, oaths, agreements, covenants, whatever we might call them, is an extremely serious matter, and there is danger in making them carelessly or imprudently. We may establish an obligation to keep them, from which we may need to be released if they have been ungodly, wrong, unwise or no longer capable of being fulfilled. In retrospect they may sound so stupid that you might feel that God would not bother with such trivialities. But remember, Satan knows all the law and if we do not live in obedience to our Lord we give the enemy an opening to mess up our lives.

However, our God is merciful; as we have said, he gives us the opportunity to turn and repent. There are verses of Scripture which deal with how to be released from vows. He will provide a way of escape. Always remember that God knows and understands your need for forgiveness and restoration and, in his love for you, he has made provision for a fresh start. Under the old covenant, he made provision for dealing with sin; repentance was to be real; sacrifices were to be offered in the manner prescribed. In the new covenant, Jesus himself is the provision. He gave his life as a sacrifice, in order that our sins might be forgiven. (See Hebrews 10:12). We received forgiveness of all our sins when we were born again. Whatever sins you may have committed up to that point, they were washed away by the blood of Jesus wholly and completely, as God's free gift to you — as you received Jesus as your Lord and Saviour. His work on the cross has set you free. Jesus defeated Satan, broke the power of sin, broke the curse, and provides the means for us to be freed from all oppression. The process I will describe here helps us to live in greater awareness of the freedom that Jesus won for us in his unique, unrepeatable sacrifice for you and me, which we received by the grace of God, through faith.

First, we ask the Holy Spirit to show us where we may have unresolved vows or agreements.

1) Then we ask Father to forgive us for any fault or action on our part that contributed to the breakdown of the marriage or marriages.

2) We then forgive our spouse for anything that they did to hurt us, or which contributed to the breakdown of the marriage.

3) We then ask Father to forgive us for breaking the vows we made and, by the sacrifice which Jesus made on the cross for us as full payment, to release us from them.

4) If there has been more than one marriage, then it is best to deal with each one separately, referring to the spouse concerned by name.

5) Should there have been any other person or persons involved in the breakdown, then we should forgive them also.

6) If we have already entered into a new marriage we need to ask Father to forgive us for doing so before we were free and clear from our previous marriage, and ask him to bless this current union.

7) Whilst doing this we need to use the sword of the Holy Spirit, the word of God, to cut ourselves free from all soul and spiritual ties still connecting us with our previous spouses, plus any other sexual

partners we may have had and with all other persons with whom we may have had sexual relations. It is also worthwhile cutting our children free from any ungodly soul and spiritual ties coming down to them through us.

8) We need to ask the Holy Spirit to come and seal all our spiritual openings and places of vulnerability.

Even if the relationships were cohabitation rather than marriages, the probability is that we have made some vows or promises —that we would always love them or be there for them, for example. These need to be dealt with in the same way. Even if the sexual encounter was simply a one-night affair, or even only a few moments of sexual intimacy, it is still necessary to ask forgiveness and be cut free from all soul and spiritual ties with everybody with whom each of the partners has had a sexual relationship. Then the same should be done in relation to everyone with whom each of those people has had sexual relationships, which might be adversely affecting the marriage relationship —until all improper vows are released and the ties cut with the sword of the Spirit.

Using similar steps, it is certainly worth asking Father to release us from any other vows, promises, oaths or covenants that we have made, and either not kept, or realise now were silly things to do. Again I refer back to the list of common factors for failure to conceive, such as saying that you would never have babies or never have anything to do with the opposite sex.

I would suggest that it is never too early to start asking the Holy Spirit to highlight any vows you may have made which have really had the same effect as cursing your own life. People say things like this: "I'll never let anyone get close to me again." "I'll never put myself in a position to be hurt like that again." "I'll never say anything again." "No one will ever see me like that again." The list is endless. Look at some of the indicators in your life now. Are you afraid to stand in front of a group of people and speak? Are you frightened to walk into a room on your own? Do you find it impossible to make a close friend? These can sometimes stem from the root of making foolish vows (but please do not assume that this is necessarily so; there can be many other possible causes of such feelings).

There can be many quite different factors in one healing. Consider this example of scoliosis. A lady came forward for prayer, who I will call Anna for this case study. The first thing she mentioned was that she had bad teeth. It transpired that this ran in the family; we would need to deal with generational problems, and make sure that she and future generations would not suffer from this problem. Then Anna told me that she had arthritis and a weakness in her bones. It had been concluded that these two problems stemmed from the fact that her mother had needed to take a particular medication during her pregnancy with Anna. I acknowledged this information when it came to light, but waited to see what the Lord still had to reveal. As she stood in front of me I was aware that Anna's shoulders were not straight, and I started on a complete alignment of her body. First the arms and shoulders were lined up, and, as I started to pray for her back, Anna mentioned that her mother had recently told her that, when she had first realised that she was pregnant with Anna, she had considered having an abortion. When her mother had given Anna this startling piece of information she also asked Anna whether she could forgive her. Anna told me that she had been able to forgive her mother, and as she did so she felt that something lifted off her. She realised then that throughout her life she had always felt rejected —and now that had gone. I suggested to Anna that it would be good if she could persuade her mother to do these things: ask the Lord to forgive her both for considering an abortion and for taking harmful medication (since, even though this was a medical prescription, we still need to be cleared for our part); then accept that she was forgiven for all that the Lord had already forgiven her, and come out from that place of guilt. All this would help to ensure that healing that was already beginning would not be lost.

I then released Anna from the curse of the abortion and rebuked the spirits of death and infirmity that had taken up residence since that time. I told them that they no longer had authority to stay. I nullified, through the sacrifice of Jesus on the tree, the curse of speaking badly of each other that had gone on through the family for generations. This seemed to have been a family trait. Then I spoke creation power to all the vertebrae down her spine, and then her pelvic area, commanding all the bones, discs, muscles and tissue to come into proper alignment without anything being trapped, and for any part which was damaged in any way to be re-created as God had originally designed. I told the spinal column to be open so that no nerve would be trapped. I commanded the marrow in the bones to make the proper, pure blood, with the correct balance of corpuscles, and told the blood to flow through her system washing out all the impurities and deposits causing the arthritis, that the bones would regenerate and be made strong. I asked the Holy Spirit to come with the oil of anointing, and to soak into all Anna's joints, bringing release. I sat Anna down in a chair and it could clearly be seen that her ankles were at least an inch out of alignment. So I commanded the hips and legs and knees to come into alignment.

As I did this, it all visibly started to happen. You could see the ankles moving. Anna said that she could feel warmth in her hips. It was only then she told me that she had scoliosis; that one of her vertebrae kept her spine bent, her ribs crooked and her legs out of alignment.

Happily, there was a medical practitioner standing near us. He offered to check Anna properly. He carried out all the checks and tests that they use to diagnose scoliosis. He had her bend forwards and observed the straightness across her hips. He checked her shoulders and whatever else was necessary. The doctor then declared that if she had had scoliosis before, she did not have it now. As he had not examined her prior to the ministry he could not confirm that she had suffered from scoliosis before. Anna was completely released, and we give God all the glory.

9

DEPRESSION, PHOBIAS
ALLERGIES AND M.E.

If you are in depression, or have some inexplicable sickness or disability, or a fear you have never been able to conquer, or a phobia, or M.E. or chronic fatigue syndrome, may I suggest that you check to see if there are any 'unpaid' vows in your life. They could be any small thing that you said and have forgotten because it seemed so trivial to you, or something that you promised God that you would do. It may have seemed a small thing to you, but to God it is a vow. Ask, and the Holy Spirit will help you to check this out.

Then it was backache, now it is depression[1]
It used to be bad backs that were the main concern for healing at meetings, and perhaps that need not surprise us as back problems are very common, but nowadays it seems as if an epidemic of depression amongst renewed Christians has taken over. It is perhaps worth noting, incidentally, that depression is a condition that touches the lives of a great many people, possibly as many as one in five of the population at some point in their lives.

My wife (who is a psychodynamic counsellor) and I are involved in counselling. Much of Dorothy's secular counselling, as is to be expected, centres around areas of depression, but the surprising thing is that there seems to be an increasing number of born again, Spirit baptised believers who are deep in the pits of depression. At our meetings at Beggars Roost, more and more of those wanting ministry claim depression or M.E. as the reason. On enquiry, the majority

155

of them turn out to be born again, baptised in the Spirit, tongues speaking, committed Christians. Why is this? How can it be?

At our meetings, and at the vast renewal meetings, the delegates sing songs of victory in Christ, marching as soldiers of Christ and of being adopted sons. Men and women who have been applauding and proclaiming victory over Satan and all his devious ways are depressed or being held back by the debilitating lethargy of M.E.

During the Christian conference/camp/rally season, hundreds of thousands of Christians sing, dance, pray and proclaim how they are moving forward, so that it seems it cannot be long before the whole of the British Isles will not only have turned to Christ but also experience revival. Yet still the ratio of Christians to the rest of the UK population continued to decline from 1975 to the 1990s. We read of thousands attending Alpha courses all over the country and the world, resulting in thousands of commitments to Christ. Yet, all too often, the results include more fodder for the miseries. I wondered and pondered and considered this puzzling observation and got nowhere, until a glimmer of light came through when I read an article on the subject of temptation.[2] Now the light started to shine and illuminate what I shall call 'victorious depression syndrome'. In his article the author told how temptation often strikes when we are in a place of peak spiritual awareness. He gave the example of the baptism of Jesus and his subsequent trials in the desert. He also mentioned that Billy Graham acknowledged that he was often sorely tempted following his most successful crusades. We know that Jesus was successful in overcoming the temptations in the desert without falling into sin. Collating the temptation stories of Jesus in the four Gospels it is seen, firstly, that Jesus is acknowledged by John as someone he felt should be baptising him rather than the other way round, whose sandals John is not fit to untie; the Lamb of God who takes away the sin of the world. Secondly, the whole of the assembled populace witnessed the heavens opening: *...and the Holy Spirit descended on him in bodily form like a dove. And a voice came from heaven: "You are my Son, whom I love; with you I am well pleased"* (Luke 3:22). This was certainly a 'peak spiritual experience' for Jesus, being acknowledged by man, the Holy Spirit and Father God. Then the Spirit drove him into the wilderness where he experienced temptations. There are many other models in both Testaments of this pattern of a spiritual high point followed by temptation. They show that sinful, fallible men do not have the same moral fibre as Jesus for whom, of course, the outcome of temptation was quite different than in all other cases, as we are shown how he resisted the temptations perfectly. As I studied the pattern I realised that there was frequently a further stage in the sequence of events, which can follow on from temptation in those who fail to totally resist it, and that is depression.

Moses was continually having high times with God and then spending days crying to him when things did not quite work out as he would have liked. (See, for example, Exodus 15:15; 15:25; 17:4.)

Saul was chosen by God, anointed by the Spirit, prophesied with the prophets, won great and mighty battles in the name of the Lord, but failed the temptations, particularly those of pride and jealousy. His actions, such as trying to pin David to the wall with a spear, and then trying to do much the same to his son Jonathan, would suggest that he went around depressed until he died in battle. (See 1 Samuel 18:11, 20:33.)

In 1 Kings 18 and 19, Elijah is the great prophet of God. He defies the priests of Baal. God acknowledges him before them and all the people, with the tremendous miracle of the burning up of the drenched sacrifice. Almost immediately afterwards he is tempted or tested by the fear of Jezebel threatening him. She does not even have to face him directly or speak to him —all she does is send him a letter, and he flees. He is so depressed that he wants to die. (See 1 Kings 19:4). And that is where so many people are today in their depression. They know that God is supreme, but they are so consumed with their own failure or fear that they feel useless that they just want to curl up and die.

There are also numerous examples of this in the New Testament. Even at the Last Supper we see two of them. All the disciples have by this time recognised Jesus as the Messiah; they have witnessed miracle after miracle, they have even driven out demons and healed in the very name of Jesus, and now he washes their feet. Even for them this is a highly emotional and spiritual time. Although Jesus warns him, Judas is immediately tested, succumbs and then goes around in depression until he commits suicide.

Then we have Peter, too, although Jesus warned him. Peter was soon tested, denying Jesus three times. Despite the resurrection and meeting with Jesus, we later see Peter wandering restlessly through a haze of self-pity. At a loss to know what to do with himself, he decides to go fishing rather than hang around in the city. Then, after protesting his love for Jesus, he is still hung up about his own standing in relation to that of John. We do not see Peter come out of his miseries until Pentecost, when his mind is so filled with the wonder of Christ that he can do nothing else all day but tell people about him. (Acts 2:14ff.)

Were the disciples suffering from victorious depression syndrome, [VDS]? Have we not all been in, or close to, this place? There we are, right on the peak, the mountain top, with Jesus. We have the victory, we have eternal life. He who is in me is greater than he who is in the world; we are invincible, and then —wham! We meet a time of testing, no matter how big or small it might be. It may be so tiny, but we miss the mark; we do not measure up as we feel we should do. For many Christians this spells failure. We are not invincible; we are not victorious; we can sing the songs, say the prayers, but the light has gone out. Darkness has come in and depression, uselessness, sadness, lethargy, tiredness soak into our minds and bodies, leeching away all the victory. I had witnessed this scenario over and over again without understanding what was happening. People often tell us that the depression started after a time of spiritual uplift. However, the temptation or testing can have been so small an issue that it was overlooked or discounted by them as being of no consequence. But it was the opening for depression. Who put out the light?

So often, in Christian circles, we hear so much about how great has been the attack of the enemy and how much suffering Satan has caused the victim. At the big rallies warnings are given that Satan is prowling and that he may devour those who fail to resist him, but we know that we are victorious, we are invincible, we are marching. Then, wham, down we go —and we blame Satan. We plead to the Lord to deliver us from this darkness. But is it necessarily Satan? Again we can look to the Scriptures for the clues. We note that it was the Spirit who led Jesus into the desert to be tempted by the devil (see Matthew 4:1).

In John 6, after great teaching from Jesus and seeing many miracles, the disciples are on the mountain with Jesus —literally a peak experience. Seeing the massive crowd coming, Jesus tests Philip by asking him where they were going to buy supplies to feed them. Philip responds with a comment about the cost. Despite all that Philip knew about Jesus it seems that still he could either not comprehend the riches that are in Christ Jesus, or not believe to receive them. In John 6:6 it says, *He asked this only to test him, for he already had in mind what he was going to do.* We can see that it is not necessarily the devil having his evil way or causing trouble, but can be very much about how we respond to God's word.

If we intend to march in victory there is no way that we can avoid going via a route that includes testing and temptation. If we are going to go forward then be assured that there is a minefield of testing and temptation just waiting to blow us into VDS. How do we get through the minefield without being blown up? Jesus did. If the temptation is straight from the devil, as it seemed to be for Jesus in the wilderness, then his example of bombproof clothing was a mind full of the Scriptures. Most of us want to argue with the problem and tell it to go away, or try and pray it away, but not Jesus. It is no good arguing with evil. Jesus simply quoted Scripture, the word of God, to Satan. But remember it needs to be the *rhema* word —that is, it needs to be the truth that God has recently spoken into us. It needs to be the truth of the living word of God at work in us.

We are reminded of how Jesus again faced a huge challenge in the Garden of Gethsemane. Things were very tough indeed, and he prayed to the Father that if the Father were willing, the 'cup' would be taken from him; but that the Father's will be done. (See Luke 22:42.)

You need to be very sure that the route map you are following for your walk is the one you have been given by God; that you are going in the direction that he wants; that you are doing the things he wants you to; and that you have not simply, in a wild burst of enthusiasm, gone charging off ahead of the blessing. Remember to seek for and follow where God is blessing, and not go running off expecting God to catch up.

So many suffering with VDS tell how they have been trying to work for God. They have done this or that and it all fell flat; their church turned them down; no one would help; everybody refused to help; the money ran out; they sold their home to capitalise the venture and now they are homeless. Now they are depressed and do not know how to get out.

Unless we know utterly that God has detailed any change in direction, we need to stay in the blessing, in the vision he first gave us. If we only *think* that some change is what God wants, then at least be a Gideon and put down a fleece. (See Judges 6:37.)

So how does one get out of VDS? There is no set formula by which we can be set free from depression, but this is an example of one way of praying which I have seen meet with success:

• Start by asking the Holy Spirit to be the guide in thinking back to what was happening at the time of the onset of the depression.
• Had there been a spiritual high point? What happened afterwards? Was there a situation of testing or temptation in which the Lord impressed some particular course of action? It may have seemed insignificant but we have to be faithful in the small things before he can trust us with the big ones.
• Was there victory over the temptation, passing of the test, or a feeling of failure followed by a sense of disaffection? Was there at first just a touch of the miseries, which without realising it darkened and darkened into depression or acute tiredness?
• Go back to the beginning and ask God to forgive you for not doing what he required.
• Speak out aloud that you have been forgiven and that you receive the forgiveness in Jesus' name.
• Speak out that you are washed clean of guilt and failure by the precious blood of Jesus.
• Loose from yourself any darkness, tiredness and depression and receive the light that is in Christ Jesus and the life-giving Holy Spirit.
• No matter how foolish it may seem to you, speak these things out loud. You are speaking to the faith that is in you, whether you feel you have any or not. The word says that you have your measure of faith. (See Romans 12:3.)
• Tell the mind to respond to the faith. Do not argue with your mind. Tell it.
• Start praising the Lord with the mind and the voice.
• Start proclaiming the truth of the gospel of Christ.
• Now move out into the victory, put the faith into action and be ready to be surprised by joy.
• Yes to renewal – no to destruction.

Let not the forward march of renewal be destroyed or held back by lack of knowledge. Now that we know about this pernicious victorious depression syndrome we can endeavour to avoid it. If we inadvertently catch it then let us recognise the symptoms quickly and start on the cure. We need to see the body of Christ on the march —but moving forward, not marching on the spot, marking time.

He came to Beggars Roost

I have perceived a possible similarity in patterns of behaviour prior to the onset of M.E. However it is not necessarily preceded by a spiritual high. For example, a man with a worldwide ministry, who had symptoms of M.E., came to the healing Centre. He had had to stop travelling and was fatigued and dispirited. The Lord prompted me to remind him that he had to get on with the new work into which God had called him. He realised that he had been holding back from doing this. As soon as he repented and complied with God's word, the M.E. left him. I know he has increased his ministry since then.

She came to Beggars Roost

Christine wrote to tell me that she had come all the way from the south of England to a service at the Centre for healing. She had M.E. Prior to coming north she had realised, after prayer and reflection, that it was all caused through stress. She was doing too many things, looking after a sick granddaughter as well as her own family. She was president of the Ladies' Inner Wheel Club. She was a 'Sailors, Soldiers, and Airmen's' family visitor. She was working on business on their own farm. As a result of all this stress she caught glandular fever from her granddaughter. Then she caught hepatitis and yellow jaundice, caused by an unknown virus. Bouts of nausea and stomach pains took her to a consultant who, after numerous blood tests, diagnosed M.E. and chronic fatigue. She wrote that she came to a healing service in June 1996 and that I asked her to repent of working through an illness and not resting. As she repented she was slain in the Spirit. When she went home she had more energy but says that she waited two weeks before writing to me because she wanted to make sure that her recovery was permanent. Her tiredness completely disappeared. As she wrote in a later letter, the M.E. was instantly healed.

A lady came to Beggars Roost in darkness and left in the light.
She wrote to me on a pretty Christmas card, with a dove flying freely on the front. *I'm free, and I'm ME. I'm pottering about under the Lord's benevolent gaze —He's really pleased with me (just because I'm me) and I'm basking in this unfamiliar feeling of being warmly approved. I feel so different —light and airy, about six inches taller and twenty years younger. I feel as if I have emerged from a dark and dreary place (the living death, as you described it so aptly) into the light. I am full of wonder at this amazing work God has done.*

I write this with such a grateful heart. Thank you for making time for me, for your warm welcome, for enfolding me, for teasing out all the disorder with patience and insight, and ministering the Lord's peace and healing to my tortured selfhood and body.

M.E., depression and fear

This man wrote to tell me about a visit that he paid to the Centre in May 1996. He told me that he had suffered from M.E. since 1988. He seemed to recover, only for it to return three years later, which resulted in more time off work. For a number of years his health was generally good, but stress would quickly bring back the symptoms. Depression came on through the fear that the M.E. would return. Prayer helped, but the fear still remained. That night in May he said that I told him that God was saying that to be healed he had to 'move on' in his relationship with God. Nothing spectacular happened that night, but over the months he realised that even when he got very tired and stressed, not only did the symptoms not return, but the fear of the illness had also gone. He did 'move on' in his relationship with Christ who showed himself to be a faithful Lord. Stephen praised the Lord and thanked him for his goodness and mercy. Now he encourages others suffering from M.E. and depression not to give up hope.

Sandra, who came to Beggars Roost a number of times, wrote:

Dear Randy and Dorothy,
Please forgive me that I have not written down the following major events that I have experienced during my visits to the healing Centre and conferences. In addition to these events, most weeks I have received inner healing for a 'broken heart' and several events during my childhood, and recently a word about a new job that God had for me.

At the conference in 1997 I received inner healing from the psychological effects of having had two car accidents (head on crashes). I was able forgive the two drivers who had crashed into my car. I am now able to drive in the dark again without fear.

When I came in August 1998 I had been in deep depression since the March, and it was so bad I was on sick leave for five months. At the start of the meeting Randy said, "Someone will be healed of depression tonight." Joan had received this word. I spoke to Joan and she told me that as she had walked past me earlier that evening she had a picture of a spider's web that was so thick that she couldn't see through it. Actually, as Joan walked past me I had my eyes closed and saw a picture of a big black hairy spider's leg with a hook on the end (like a barbed hook). As Joan walked past me the picture was squashed, and as it was so vivid to me I felt that I had been squashed, and I crunched up. Joan prayed for me and the depression lifted. I knew I would be healed that day. I had watched Benny Hinn on TV that morning and when he said this is your day for healing I knew that I would be healed that day. The following week I went to see my counsellor, who discharged me from her caseload, as I was better (healed).

Regards, Sandra

The curse of empathy

My dear friends The Reverend Tom Jewett and his wife, Anne, taught me about the dangers of empathy and how so many ministers and even whole churches can be virtually wiped out by wrong thinking and practice. From all I have seen since Tom pointed it out to me, empathy can be a curse to those involved in caring ministries. Generally in society, to be able to empathise with people or situations is hailed as a great virtue. Counsellors are urged to empathise with their clients so that they can really understand the problems and help the client move forward. Sadly, so often exactly the opposite takes place and in time the counsellor becomes worn out, burned out, sick and the client is still in trouble. Empathy has been defined as the power of understanding and imaginatively entering into another person's feelings. This is similar in meaning to 'identification' or incorporating aspects of the other's personality into your own. But God made each of us an individual person. Personality is the sum total of all that makes you a unique individual. It is very dangerous, and most surely against God's will, for us to endeavour to incorporate aspects of someone else's identity into our own.

In his three years of ministry, we do not read of Jesus trying to become part of someone else. We are told, though, how Jesus showed compassion. Not until the cross does he take others' hurts, sickness or trouble onto himself. We should all minister compassionately. The quality of compassion is altogether different from empathy. It can include feelings of distress and pity for the suffering of the other person; it is always full of love, centring on the true need of the person, and their value. Showing compassion is an entirely worthy emotion. Compassion motivates us to move out to help. But empathy is taking into ourselves something that is not ours to take, and is disabling rather than motivating. When somebody is in trouble and in a deep hole, it does not help to get in the hole with him or her. We need to stand on the side and find a way to pull or encourage them out. When someone is sick, it is of no assistance to them if we become part of the sickness. We then have two people who are sick and need help.

Again this is not merely splitting hairs. In fact there is an even wider need to distinguish compassion from empathy. During the three years of his earthly ministry, Jesus did not empathise. Jesus did not take problems into himself until the proper time set by Father God. Then Jesus took all sickness and sin, for the whole world, into himself on the cross. It was so awful and disfiguring that God had to make the world completely dark, so that no man could see the horror of all that was happening during those hours. We are told that Jesus did this once for all. If Jesus did it once for all, then we have no mandate to attempt to do it again. To want to try and feel someone else's pain is like saying to Jesus that what he did was not sufficient —that he failed, so now we must do it. But man cannot improve on anything Jesus has already done. Our job is to stand alongside hurting people in prayer and help them put that pain back on the cross where Jesus already dealt with it. Father God once showed me very vividly that when I held on to sin or sickness, it was as if I was putting Jesus back on the cross. He has already dealt with it, and has risen so that we can be free.

Empathy is in a very different league from words of knowledge. What do I mean by linking empathy with words of knowledge? Sometimes the Holy Spirit leads in different ways. Sometimes words of knowledge can be just that! —words, which we hear, or see, or just simply 'know that we know' about a situation. We looked at this issue in chapter six. Sometimes we see pictures. However, sometimes we can feel a pain or a niggle or some sort of sensation in part of our bodies and we know that this is alerting us to a situation that is troubling someone. This can take many forms. For instance, in chapter one I mentioned the little lady in East Berlin and the time when I could feel all the desolation and coldness and loneliness inside her.

My friend Scott Edgar, from South Carolina, contacted me at one time because he was getting very concerned. Even walking through the mall he was feeling the hurts and pains, physical and emotional, of people as they passed by. This was proving difficult to manage and was making life very uncomfortable for him. He was not sure what to do with it all and wondered whether he should he take the pains himself. I explained to him the healing ministry can be a hard and messy business, involving as it does the depths of people's misery. But to take these things into himself would be to try to do what Jesus already has done for us on the cross.

These types of experience can be God's way of alerting us to our need to intercede. It is not that we should take the pain ourselves but that in intercession we lift it up, off them and off ourselves, on to the cross where it has been dealt with. The pain and hurt is not our cross to bear, but the place of intercession is where Jesus wants us to be with him. Remember that God has seated us in the heavenly realms with Christ Jesus. (See Ephesians 2:6.) And he intercedes for us continually. We are praying for others from the throne room of God. Here are two examples of how dangerous empathy can be.

A minister's wife came to Beggars Roost
Forgiving the church and those in authority

A lady came to a Thursday evening service. She had arthritis in her hips and it was getting worse and worse. Even though experience has shown us that unforgiveness, anger and resentment are so frequently the bitter roots of arthritic and associated problems, one cannot just assume this. We must always come to Father in prayer and ask the Holy Spirit to lead us. I knew that the lady was the wife of a clergyman, but when I said to her that she had to forgive the bishop and the church I was somewhat taken aback myself. Out flooded the resentment. She felt that the bishop and church authorities had not treated her husband well or fairly. Although he took it all calmly and in his stride she had empathised completely with each ensuing situation. She felt every wrong action, every harsh word and bad decision made against him; she had taken them into herself.

I explained the crippling reaction that unforgiveness, anger and resentment can have – physically, mentally and spiritually – and how, in taking into herself all the hurts being poured out upon her husband, she was in effect taking over the role of Jesus. He did it once and for all on the cross and then said it is finished. She asked the Lord to forgive her, as she forgave the church and all the authorities.

She phoned me on the Saturday evening to say that she and her husband had walked six or seven miles in the Cheviot hills. She phoned the following week to tell how she had been to a swimming pool and swum many lengths. After swimming the lengths, she and her husband had again been walking in the hills. She did all this exercise without pain or stiffness in her hips.

I asked her to write and tell me how she had been healed but she would not do this. Many months later I discovered the reason: she was due to see the consultant at the hospital in the following January and wanted his authentication of her healing. She wrote to me the following letter on the 18th January 1997.

Dear Randy,

When I came to the Centre on July 11th 1996, I asked for prayer for healing. I had had problems with an arthritic hip for nearly three years. It was steadily worsening and I was taking at least six painkillers a day, just to keep moving —stairs were a real problem. I had seen a consultant earlier in the day and he had prescribed anti inflammatory drugs to be taken with the painkillers, to try to postpone a hip operation for as long as possible. He also said I must use a walking stick.

Praise the Lord, since being prayed for I have needed no medication at all, and have been able to enjoy walking and swimming again. I've even been hill walking several times.

I had a follow up appointment with the consultant on January 9th and he thinks further appointments are unnecessary.

I really do thank Jesus for yet another demonstration of his love and power, and thank you too, for your ministry.

A priest brought his parishioners to Beggars Roost

A couple came with their priest. Let us call them Janet and John. Janet had inoperable tumours on the brain. We asked the Holy Spirit to lead as we prayed; Dorothy and I understood that this was spiritually based and that we needed to work from there.

Janet started to tell us their story. It was apparent that she loved John deeply and looked upon him as the knight in shining armour who had rescued her from the awful life that she had led at home. We saw that it went even deeper than that: John was her life now. She idolised her husband and certainly put him before God. Both she and John believed God and were sometime churchgoers, but there was not yet any depth in their relationship with Jesus.

John was a stocky, thick set, heavily muscled man. Even through the suit that he wore one could see the muscles underneath. He told us that he was a doorman and bouncer at the night clubs. He also told us that he was a kick-boxer. He was very strong and brushed off all the knocks he took, but Janet did not. His life was so much part of her life that she lived her life through this man whom she loved above all else. She could not brush off all the blows that he took but took them into herself. She felt every blow. She had to stop going to the fights because it was too painful for her to watch. She used to stay at home, but then in her imagination she took all the blows into herself to prevent John being hurt. All the time, she worried for his safety and she empathised through every fight. The art of kick-boxing is to be able to kick high to the opponent's head. She took all those blows to the head herself and this seemed to be the source of the tumours.

We had sensed that this was a spiritual problem and so asked John about the spiritual side of his sport. He readily acknowledged this and told us how the training was more a series of spiritual exercises than it was physical. He explained to us that no man can be so physically strong or his hands so naturally hard that he can chop through bricks or thick blocks of wood with his bare hands. He knew that this power was the spiritual dimension to the sport.

We told them about the Holy Spirit, and how we should not be having connection with any spirits or deity other than Father God, our Lord Jesus Christ and the Holy Spirit; and that the only way to God was through Jesus. To put anything else before God is counted in the Bible as idolatry. Janet and John listened intently. When the idea was suggested, John readily agreed to renounce all his connection with anything other than the Holy Spirit; he asked forgiveness for involvement with the occult through the martial art of kick-boxing and promised that he would immediately give it up and sever any connection with it. They both asked Jesus to be Lord in their lives and we cut them both free from any soul and spiritual ties with the occult. Janet then asked the Lord to forgive her for idolising John and putting him before Jesus; also for empathising and taking all the blows into herself.

They went off home and, although we had no more direct contact with them ourselves, their priest sent reports from time to time that they were doing well.

Addictions and allergies

An email arrived, which said this:

I have been a compulsive eater since I was a small child and as a result of being sexually abused by my brother I would eat large quantities of food at a time —cakes, cookies, chips, whatever I could get to eat, until I was stuffed and sick. I would agonise about my weight and my body. It was an endless, painful cycle that years of therapy and prayer could not seem to break. Dorothy prayed with me about my compulsive eating. Ever since the night she prayed I have not overeaten, nor had any desire to overeat. I had been to therapists, to 12 step groups, to ministers, to conferences —all trying to figure out how to break out of this painful cycle. I had even concluded that overeating was my thorn in the flesh.
The Lord has healed me.
Thanks be to God.

We were in Hitchin

Colin became a very close friend of mine, but not before this particular night when we had been invited to his house for dinner. He was not well disposed towards us because, although Colin was a well-churched Baptist, he was not at all in favour of 'charismatics' which he knew us to be.

After dinner we were sitting talking and Colin sneezed a number of times. He explained that he had an allergy to cats. The Lord alerted me to an opening and to the fact that this allergy had not been with him since childhood. I suggested to Colin that this reaction to cats was possibly not through the normally expected source of allergies but that it could have been acquired in some other way. I asked him to think back to something that occurred just prior to the first onset of the sneezing. Colin very kindly agreed to allow his mind to look back through time, and silently I asked the Holy Spirit to highlight for him what had occurred. He remembered how he had been driving home one dark night and, as he turned the corner into the close where they lived, a cat had suddenly run into the road. Colin had been unable to stop in time and had run over the cat, killing it. It had in no way been his fault. It seemed to me that he was suffering from guilt, remorse and unforgiveness of himself. I explained this to him and he listened. Not only did he listen, he agreed to pray to release himself from guilt and to accept forgiveness of all that the Lord had already forgiven him for, and to say sorry to God for having held it all this time. We cut the bonds of guilt from him and he was immediately set free. The presence of a cat was never again able to make him sneeze. It also opened the way for further meetings. He came with me to FGBMFI dinners. He became my dear friend and the founding president of the Hitchin Chapter of the FGBMFI.

Colin died of colon cancer some years ago, still in his prime with so much still to give, and I just yearn to be able to move so far into the anointing and the presence of Jesus within me that none of my friends will die untimely deaths.

Notes
[1] Parts of the section on VDS are based on an article first published in *Renewal*, Issue 246, November 1996.
Refer now to: www.christianitymagazine.co.uk
[2] By Canon Mark Pearson, writing in the newsletter of the Institute for Christian Renewal.

10

CANCERS AND OTHER DISORDERS

These are diseases which just do not get healed without treatment. Even with treatment there is no medical cure for some of them. Medical treatment can often help alleviate the symptoms or enable the sufferer to cope with the effects of the disease. However nothing is impossible to our God. I stand in awe at the wonderful things that the authority of Jesus in the power and presence of his Holy Spirit can do. As I have tried to emphasise right through this book, the commission to heal and therefore the authority to heal was given by Jesus to his body, the church. A large part of the vision that he gave me was to encourage and enable his people to move out and heal the sick. When Jesus is present then the power to heal is present.

The power of his presence

My friend Scott Edgar emailed me from South Carolina to say that he had been reading Luke 5:17 and it seemed to him that the healing gift appears to be Spirit-driven. He wrote, *I read the other day in Luke 5:17, 'And the power of the Lord was present for him to heal the sick' —which I interpreted as, "the power" has to be present to heal the sick. Any thoughts?* It did make me think. This is how I replied: In some way I would say that you are right that the power of God has to be present to heal. But the power comes with the anointing. The anointing comes with baptism in the Holy Spirit, the receiving of the power from on high. We recall how the Holy Spirit descended on Jesus at the side of the Jordan. He then went through his time of testing, as we have to do. We learn from Luke 4:14 that he returned to Galilee in the power of the Spirit and started preaching the word. He entered the synagogue and we learn of his fulfilment of the prophecy in Isaiah 61:2. We read in Isaiah 10:27 that the anointing breaks the yoke. The anointing breaks bondage to the oppressor. If we look back again at Luke 5:17 we see that Jesus was teaching —preaching the word. Healing, life, health, all the issues of life itself, are in the word of God. Life is in the word. Jesus is the Word. Jesus is the life. When the Lord is present, the Word is present. When we preach the Word in the power of the Spirit then power is present. The verse shows that: Jesus did not have to ask for the power to heal; he did not have to seek for the power to heal; where Jesus was, the power to heal was present. That is still true today. When we look further at who was there we find that there were Pharisees and teachers from every village in Galilee, Judea and Jerusalem. This was a big meeting, perhaps some conspiracy to try to catch him out. Those men were not there to sit at his feet in order to receive the word as he was teaching. The Pharisees and the lawyers were there to judge and condemn. They did not have little faith, not even mere absence of faith; rather, they exhibited what we might call 'negative' faith. They were there to undermine or destroy anything Jesus did. We know from another passage, probably slightly earlier in Jesus' ministry, what happened when there was little faith present. On that occasion there were no miracles and only a few were healed. (See Mark 6:5f., Matthew 13:58.)

Once I asked the Lord what was happening on the occasion that there were no miracles and few healed, because we read elsewhere that Jesus healed all that came to him. (See Matthew 12:15 et al). The impression I had was that not many were healed because they did not come to him. They did not come to hear him teach. Not many had the sense to come to him in his home place. They probably gossiped amongst themselves about the fact that this was just the young fellow that they had seen growing up as the son of Mary and Joseph the carpenter and about his unusual birth. Most people know what small town gossip can be like and have possibly suffered at the hand of it. So the few who were healed would have been the only ones that came to hear him, or went to the meetings, or asked for his help.

At all times we must remember who has the power to heal. It is not us, it is Jesus. It is his authority in which we minister. When we

172

minister the word in faith, then Jesus is present. And when Jesus is present so is the power to heal. So be encouraged by this verse, not discouraged. When and where we go in Jesus' name, we go under the anointing of the Holy Spirit. Then, no matter who else is there, the power to heal is present. And as we look at the power in the word more closely, we find it is *dunamis*, MIGHTY POWER.

When we come to consider the 'gifts of healings' in 1 Corinthians 12:9 we must strongly remind ourselves that these gifts do not provide divine healers but divine healings. The gifts are the manifestation of the Holy Spirit. He owns the gifts. He gives gifts of healings to believers as he sees that they have need to have them demonstrated as flowing from his infilling. We need to stress that we see that this is not a gift given only to exceptional ministers, who the sick need to seek out in order to receive God's healing. No, it is through all those who believe that he can manifest his grace, power and will. Therefore when we look at so many of these wonderful stories of healing in this book we see that it is the members of the congregations who are laying on hands and speaking healing into peoples lives, not just Dorothy and myself.

Healed of cancer; Carole Pagnotto's story

Following one of our missions we received this article, which was published in the church magazine. Again it was a member of their prayer team who directly ministered; neither Dorothy nor I was personally involved in praying with the lady. But we know that, as we proclaim the truth about the kingdom, the presence of Jesus and his anointing power to heal will fill the room.

Five months ago I had a mammogram done and it showed that I had a spot on my left breast. Several more mammograms were done at this time and I was told that I would be watched and should have another one done in six months.

I received a call from my doctor telling me that she wanted me to have a follow up mammogram done ASAP, and an appointment was set for me to have the procedure done. At that time again several mammograms were done and all showed the same spot in the same location. I was told that the radiologist would study the films for comparison and they would get back to me. Needless to say I was more than a little worried and stressed. Prayer was needed and my husband and I were looking forward to the Vickers healing mission that would be held the following Friday, Saturday and Sunday. During the Friday services I asked for prayer, and a lady by the name of Diane came and prayed for me. We went to the back of the hall during the lady's prayer for my healing; she named the spot as cancer and said that I would be OK. I wanted to put my hand over her mouth and tell her no, no, this wasn't cancer. In her prayers at one point she said that she felt the Lord was telling her that my husband and I had not been together very long. I told her that we had been married for three months. She said the Lord was not going to separate us and that he had work for my husband and me to do. That was so comforting!

She continued to pray and then she said that she felt the Lord was also telling her that my husband and I had made a pact with him (which we had) and that he was honouring that pact, and that pact was that there were not two of us in our marriage, but that there were three of us: Jesus, my husband and me. The lady then told me about her experience as a cancer patient and again assured me that I would be OK. We left feeling confident that all was in God's hands and that no matter what, with his help I would deal with it.

I received a call telling me that the spot was "different" and that I had to go in for a sonogram at 10:40 the next morning. My doctor called me and told me that my husband should be with me; that they would do the sonogram and then a biopsy. She sounded very ominous but, of course, told me not to worry! Ha! I immediately got on the internet to all my wonderful sisters in Christ, to start praying, and in no time I felt bathed in prayer.

On our way to the hospital, my husband said he knew that I was OK and we both assured each other that there was nothing to worry about. Everything was in the hands of our Saviour, the Great Physician and we knew that there was nothing too difficult for him.

When the technician started the sonogram, I was looking at the monitor, looking for the spot, and I couldn't see it and neither could she! Joe was standing behind her with tears in his eyes and silently giving a cheer sign as she kept saying that this was all clear and that she was anxious to have the radiologist see her results. She was gone about 15 minutes and that gave Joe and me time to pray and praise the Lord for his faithfulness. When she arrived back in the room, she said the doctor wanted a full sonogram done to the entire left side. Again, during the procedure, she kept telling us that there was

NOTHING THERE and the three of us were laughing as we gave glory to God. She gave this report to the doctor and he had her come in and tell me that I was just fine, and to go home!

My doctor called me later in the day and she was just incredulous! I told her this was the power of prayer and she readily agreed! Now all I need to do is to return for another mammogram in six months. I think I will be able to handle that.

We are so grateful and thankful for this healing, and my husband and I give all the honour, praise and glory to our Lord Jesus Christ, Jehovah Rapha, our healer; Jehovah Jirah, our provider and El Shaddai, the all-sufficient One!

And another email:

I heard a wonderful praise report last night. You prayed with my friend. She has gone through cancer surgery this year, and chemo. One side effect from the chemo has been some hearing loss. After you prayed for her, one ear completely cleared up and, in the days following, the other ear cleared up. She said she continues to have NO problem. She is praising the Lord and thanking you for your prayers. She does ask your prayers for surgery she is scheduled for in the morning. Due to the cancer a large portion of her lung was removed. She continues to have fluid in the lungs. They are performing a surgery where they rough up the sides of the lungs and then pull the sides together and adhesions form. We prayed with her last night for immediate regeneration and healing, a long peace, etc. I know she would welcome your prayers.

Pat was brought to Beggars Roost

This is Pat Hardy's story of defeating cancer, as she emailed it to me. The first night that she came to Beggars Roost was a horrible, cold, snowy night. The roads were treacherous, but Pam Pritchard, who is one of our ministry team, was very anxious that her friend might die. The prognosis was very grim, and Pat was so ill and desperate that in spite of all the weather warnings on the radio and television, not to travel unless essential, they braved the elements and the Lord kept them safe from harm. Pat came to the Centre and received prayer, and on the way back home both she and Pam agreed that they felt God's amazing peace.

Pam lived twenty miles away from Pat, and after dropping Pat at her home she realised that the snow was deep and drifting, and she wondered how she could get home that night. As she came away from Pat's and skidded towards the main road, a snowplough came along going in her direction so she tucked in behind it. For me we now enter the area of the miraculous. The two ladies not only live in widely separated different council districts, they live in entirely different counties. In my experience, never the twain shall meet. One council never clears the roads of another. One county does not use its resources in another county, but this snowplough carried on through all the boundaries in exactly the direction that Pam needed. She was able to safely follow it all the way home to her village. She was met by her husband on the drive, as he had rushed out to greet her the moment he had seen the headlights. He had been very worried.

Later on in the same week, Pat rang Pam to tell her that the bleeding had stopped and her blood count had come up. Her healing had started and is now complete. [That preface to the story was actually edited and amended for me by Pam herself.] This is Pat's story:

Hi Randy,

You have my permission to use this story in any publication or work you wish to use it in. I first visited Beggars Roost healing Centre, Stocksfield in February 2001. I was in no fit state to get there but my friend and former colleague Pam had been there and had received an amazing healing. She very much wanted me to have the same and, out of love, came through snow and ice to get me and take me to the Thursday healing service.

I had just had an extensive operation to remove ovarian tumours and was one treatment into a course of chemotherapy. The tumours were malignant and very advanced. The chemotherapy was to destroy any remaining small cells and any remaining infected tissue. At the time of my first visit my CA125, a cancer marker in the blood, was over 250. Normal levels in any female range between 0 and 35 so I was well over my acceptable level.

In hospital I had been very upset at the diagnosis, and the prognosis was not particularly helpful either. I was told repeatedly that I would be lucky to live beyond five more years, and that the cancer would return. There was a one in ten chance that I would survive. I had a fabulous nurse who was so positive, but I knew that this illness was really testing my faith. I felt empty and lost. There was nothing I could do to change this situation, but I knew that God could change it. I also knew that this did not always happen, and my prayers varied from wanting to be there for my children to wanting God to give me the strength to cope.

When I arrived at the Centre I remember wanting the service to end so that we could get to the prayer bit. I was desperate to hear from God. Randy came to me and began to pray. I think I was the only person he prayed with that night. I was very scared; I think we all are when we know we are in the presence of God, and Randy began to pray. He made me feel that it was not my fault that I had cancer. He prayed about any links with cancer in my family. This amazed me as at that time I had only told my husband that I was scared because I was 41 and my Mum had died aged 41 from cancer. My Dad had also died when he was 41, from a pulmonary embolism. Here was Randy praying for the very thing I feared. He prayed for all fear to go. He prayed in such a loving and gentle way, and I felt that God was showing me his love, respect and honour for me. Randy also prayed against curses, and then he prayed for cleansing and anointed my right ear, thumb and big toe. I was very puzzled by that, but knew that the Holy Spirit was leading Randy in his prayers. There were other things that spoke into my heart and told me that God was there right in the core of all of it, and that just because I did not understand it did not mean that God was not working.

Observations from Randy:

(a) We have found that when a medical diagnosis is spoken over a patient it can have the same effect as cursing someone. Without even being conscious of it most people accept the diagnosis as defining who or what they are, and they personally 'own' it. People tend to say such things as 'I have cancer'; 'My cancer is terminal'; 'My son is autistic.' They do not just say it, they actually believe it. How should we handle this? Well, in the case of our granddaughter Lucy, who was diagnosed at birth as being affected by Downs Syndrome, that is the way in which we accepted it, as affecting her. We are not in denial of the diagnosis, we simply will not give the diagnosis the right and authority to define and own Lucy. We do not think or refer to Lucy as being a Downs baby, or as having Downs Syndrome. The diagnosis, and knowing some of the effects that this syndrome can have on the person, gives us an indication of the ways in which we have to pray to see her body accept the healing. We live in the expectation of seeing Lucy grow up as a normal girl, and as the various symptoms show themselves we pray accordingly.

(b) Jesus became a curse for us, so that even the Gentiles would receive the blessing and receive the promise of the Spirit through faith. (Galatians 3:13f.) Therefore, in the case of Pat I took the authority in Jesus' name, to release the power of the curse from her and declare it null and void. So often, too, we have found that when a doctor proclaims a diagnosis over a patient, without even being conscious of it, a person can become fearful. Fear, the Scriptures tell us, does not come from God. We are admonished so many times in the Bible not to be anxious. This may seem a hard thing to say but, with the best will in the world, fear is a sin. However, as can be seen from the way in which Pat tells the story, we are very gentle with the way we use language when ministering. We do not lay any further burdens on those who are very tired and weary from carrying the weight of their sickness. As we have seen, it is the anointing that breaks the yoke that binds them. Fear shows where we do not trust God. (I am not talking about the sort of 'fear' that is there to save us from harm, such as fearing to stick your hand into a hot fire because you know it will burn, or which is there to stop us doing some other foolhardy thing. I do not call that fear. I call that common sense.)

(c) This is not necessarily a spirit of fear, and we know that if there is one, God did not give it to us. (See 2 Timothy 1:7.) I think that this is our soulish reaction to the news of the diagnosis, and as such can be released through repentance and forgiveness.

(d) But so often in the case of the diagnoses of illnesses or diseases which can be terminal, along with the fear we can open ourselves to a spirit of death. With Father God's forgiveness comes the authority for deliverance from the spirit of death.

(e) As will be noticed in Pat's description of the events, as the Lord led me, I also dealt with wrong soul ties and generational problems.

(f) Pat mentions my anointing her right ear, thumb and big toe. I was actually using the practice of first the blood and then the oil, following the ritual of cleansing that is laid out in Leviticus 14:12–20. As we need no other sacrifice than Jesus and the blood that he shed on the cross, I symbolically put the blood of Christ on the tip or lobe of Pat's right ear, then on the thumb of her right hand, then on the big toe of her right foot. The Scriptures tell us that the priest then used to take some of the special oil for anointing and put it on top of the blood on the tip of the ear, the thumb and the big toe. We can use oil which has been blessed. However, as the oil is a symbol of the anointing of the Holy Spirit, in the absence of oil we can ask the Holy Spirit to come as the oil of anointing and cover the blood, and we symbolically apply it to the ear, the thumb and the big toe. For further information on this way of ministering I recommend that you buy what I think is the best ever reference book written about healing, *The Good News that Nobody Wanted to Know* (details at the end of chapter 5 above.)

Pat continues: *I remembered that I had been given a prophecy in hospital, which said that I was going to go through the dark places but that Jesus and me were going together over boulders and through the valley, and that at the end of the healing many would look at me and see God's work. I thought that this was a very nice sentiment but that it was not much help to me except that I made myself picture it whenever I felt my thoughts becoming black. There was a real battle going on for my mind.*

Observation from Randy: Pat actually came back to the Centre on the following Thursday night. She looked very different from the figure at death's door who had been with us the previous week. She stood and gave her testimony of how she had been healed the week before. It was obvious that the fear and the spirit of death had gone from her. Although it would be some time before science would confirm her healing, Pat had started to live in the assurance of what Jesus had done.

Pat continues:

Within a month the cancer marker in my blood was down to under 10, and was well within the normal range for a healthy adult. In this time I never caught a cold or illness and I continued with my chemotherapy until the end of the course. At the end of the course my CA125 was 4. I was so happy.

Returning to work and to my family made me appreciate every single day was a gift from God, and that I had a responsibility to look after the body he had given me. Before my illness I was a slave to stress. I would stay up all night doing work, and was not eating correctly or exercising at all. I was overworked and did not believe that God wanted me to have some fun in my life. I took the stance that if I was asked to do something then I would do it because it must be from God. I had people calling on me for prayer and ministry at any time of day or night and would drop what I was doing to try and help them. I felt such a failure when I had cancer. My church was totally gobsmacked! They could not believe that I could be ill. To them I was too close to God to become ill. It really rocked their faith and they petitioned God for me and showed me such amazing love in a million very practical ways. I remember that two people brought me perfume and I was really touched because that was something I could appreciate. I had been a prolific reader but there was nothing I could keep my mind on. Chocolates and fruit did not appeal as I had such problems with the taste of food due to my chemo. I also had problems with my feet and had severe itching and pain in them following chemo. I was able to face the other side effects, but this would reduce me to tears it was so intensely painful. Looking back, I can see that my feet were a problem when I tried to do too much instead of resting.

I learned a lot about healthy eating and the importance of a healthy lifestyle, and that God wanted us to be healthy and have balance in our lives. I was so pleased that I was well, and managed to stay well for two years. Then the unbelievable happened: once again my cancer marker went up and was over 500. I thought that it was a mistake. Cancer could not be active again. I was well and did not have any symptoms. I had to go to hospital and have a series of scans and tests. They indicated that there was a range of tiny active cells and that there was no way surgery was an option. There was no cure for this cancer and, while chemotherapy could extend my life expectancy, there were decisions to be made about the quality of my life in that time. As long as I had no symptoms the medical advice was that it would be okay for me not to have treatment until symptoms occurred. It was up to me.

Observation from Randy: At this stage her friend Pam phoned me. What should they do? How could they pray? Both of them were frightened by this second onslaught of cancer. It appeared that they were both more frightened of this second diagnosis than when Pat had first come to the Centre with no hope and a prognosis of only five years to live at best. Again, fear is the signal that there are places within us that do not trust the Lord. As we bring these to him and receive his forgiveness, a blessing of his peace, which is incomprehensible in the light of the circumstances, pervades our very being with hope and strength and assurance. Pam and I prayed together on the phone, and she received peace about the situation.

Pam then prayed in a similar manner with Pat.

Pat continues:

I read a book given to me by Dorothy Vickers called 'Healed of Cancer', by Dodi Osteen. This lady was healed by knowing healing scriptures, and used Scripture every day in the very real battle for her mind and for her life. I had just been on a course at work called 'Investment in Excellence', and the emphasis was on the fact that how we think affects chemicals in our body. As I read the book given to me, the two seemed to come together and I decided to get well. I would fix my eyes on Christ and, whatever the battle going on around me, I would ignore it and focus on him alone.

Over the summer of 2003 I read that book again and again, highlighting verses in my Bible and putting post-it notes with verses on around my house. I found those in the book and added others that were meaningful to me. In August, while on holiday on the Isle of Wight, I was admitted to hospital as my abdomen had filled with fluid due to active cells. They drained several litres of liquid from me and I was told to make peace with my God if I had a faith.

When I returned, I decided that I would go for further chemo. Up until then I had wanted to have the faith of Dodi Osteen and just trust God for my healing. As soon as I decided to go for chemo I felt that God was saying it was the right thing to do. During this time I was far more careful with my body and learned to really shout at the devil to get his hands off my health. I also learned a new and deeper way to pray and knew that God was changing me. As Christmas drew near, I had a sudden feeling that I was not going to have the last of my chemo. My final treatment was due on Christmas Eve and I knew that God was going to give me Christmas without sickness and that I would not have any more chemo. My blood count was so low it was not safe for me to have that last dose of chemo. My blood did not recover until it got to a time when it would not be worthwhile giving me that last treatment.

I have been well ever since. There are times when my mind wanders to 'what-ifs', but then I use the Bible verses to combat my thoughts and to refocus on the truth of God's word instead of feelings and fears. I feel I am standing on a rock.

Prior to my illness I had asked God about ordination as I had felt his call and had had that confirmed. Through my illness I have had many and increasing confirmations that this is God's will for me.

When Randy prayed for me and anointed my right ear, thumb and toe, that was the cleansing of a priest from Leviticus 8:22–24.

Observation from Randy: When I applied the blood and the oil I was thinking of Leviticus 14, where it was used for cleansing the sick, but perhaps I was also being prophetic in that, as Pat indicates, the same ritual was used in preparing a man for priesthood.

Pat continues:

Over and over again, God has confirmed that this is the direction he wants me to take, and since deciding to follow this call I have had so many confirmations from others. I do not know or understand all that the last four years have been about, but I have learned so much about God being at work in what might appear to be messy situations and that we do not always have all of the answers.

Love and appreciation in our Lord, Pat

We went to Laredo, Texas

Whilst we were in Laredo, a female member of the Presbyterian church asked us to pray for her friend in hospital with cancer in San Antonio, and if possible to visit her when we reached there. The lady, Pastor Dale Youngs and the church were already praying. By the time we reached San Antonio they had sent the sick lady home from hospital, as there was nothing more that they could do, so we could not visit. Dorothy phoned her home though and spoke with her husband every afternoon that we were over in the USA, and we all prayed. Later we received this email from the lady in the church.

Subject: Miraculous healing

Well, I can hardly contain myself!!!! Please feel the ultimate joy I have through the 'mails'...........

SHE IS CANCER-FREE!! The last MRI revealed NO cancer in her pancreas, NO cancer in her liver, NO cancer in her kidneys! The doc assured her that she was NOT going to die! PRAISE GOD for his miracle, and for her testimony that will continue to change many people. I stood up in church today and relayed this news while jumping up and down and crying —she is in the 2% of people with this type of cancer who survive. God obviously has a mighty purpose for her. Please keep up your prayers for her stamina and physical strength to improve —she has literally been bed-ridden since June 24th and has great difficulty walking. Thanks, prayer warriors, for keeping the faith. Isn't God just so very, very good? Ephesians 2:8 says... 'for you have been healed by grace, through faith, but it is not through yourself, but from God!' AMEN.

We went to Durham: an example of distant healing by proxy

One winter's evening I was asked to speak at an FGBMFI dinner in Durham. After speaking, I led a time of ministry for any who wanted prayer. A woman came forward and told me about her niece who lived in Dublin. The niece was ill with cancer and her aunt wondered whether it would be permissible to pray for her as she was many miles away. I assured her that we could do this. At the dinner that night there was a young lady who was about the same age as the niece. I asked her whether she would be willing to come forward and let me lay hands on her in proxy for the young girl who was ill. She readily agreed to this. I then prayed in the normal way, commanding the sick girl's body to come into agreement with the Lord's will that she be healed. I cursed the cancer, commanding it to shrivel and die and disappear completely. I commanded the spirit of death accompanying the cancer to leave the girl. When I saw the uncle and aunt again a long time after that night they told me how they had gone to the wedding of their niece in Dublin in the summer, and how she had been completely well without any sign of cancer or sickness.

We went to Alamo Heights Methodist Church

One of our favourite places to teach and minister is at Alamo Heights Methodist Church in San Antonio, Texas. Apart from the fact that it gives us the chance to stay with our great friends Nora and Bob Scott, we get to meet with so many wonderful Christians to whom I feel very close. Nora and Bob introduced us to their senior pastor David McNitzky, and he gave his permission for me to speak at one of their small Wednesday night meetings in the prayer chapel. I think David felt that I could not do too much harm at that one service. Praise the Lord that Jesus quietly ministered to quite a number of people. I remember one young man, who just happened to be in town that night visiting with his folks, was healed from an athletic injury. His healing encouraged others to receive. I feel a significant turning point for the church that night was that one of the senior members of the church had come. He came very sceptical about us, and fairly 'anti' the whole idea of healing. God is so gracious. I did not know about his scepticism, and God gave me a word of wisdom for the man, which I was able to speak to him without anyone else hearing. Some months later he came to me and told me just how opposed he had been to the prospect of our ministering in his church. However he knew that no one else in the church could have had any knowledge whatsoever of the personal things that I had spoken to him. He was then certain that it could only have come from God, and his whole attitude was turned around.

Some time later, when corresponding with David McNitzky, he wrote to me about that night:

God's timing as always is amazing. I received your note when I got home from teaching a lesson on 'The Person, Presence and Power of the Holy Spirit'. I told them about that evening in the Garden Chapel. I recall saying to a sceptical member behind me in a pew, "I've learned to not get in the way when God is moving." He then, minutes later, went forward to you.

The events of that evening led on to our leading a retreat and a week of teaching at Alamo Heights a year or so later, when Will Bellamy's release from MS was started. But I did not hear his story until 2004 when Dorothy and I travelled over to San Antonio to work with the Order of St Luke, to lead a healing mission which was to be centred at this same church.

Not long before we were due to travel I needed urgent dental work, which involved digging out one of my wisdom teeth and a couple of others. This left me with stitches in my gums, my face frozen down the left side, including my lip. Infection set into the gums and I had ulcers in my mouth. On the evening before leaving, this infection spread to the urinary tract, involving rapid dashes to the bathroom at least every thirty minutes. We needed to be at the airport on the Monday morning before 6 a.m. to fly, first, to Amsterdam, then to Memphis, and finally on to San Antonio. I dared not eat or drink for nine hours, from Amsterdam to Memphis. I had time to remind God that this was supposed to be a healing mission, and ask him what sense did it make, for me to be travelling to pray for others to be healed, when I was such a mess. For almost nine hours God stayed silent. Then the only thing that I understood him to say to me was that he wanted me travelling until I was 85 years of age.

On such occasions, when we are physically experiencing pain and illness, it may seem foolish to attempt to stay in that place of peace and assurance; of knowing that it is the nature and will of God to heal; and that by his stripes we are healed. Our body and soul are screeching out that this cannot be true, seeming to say, *'Just look at yourself—you are ill. How can it be true that you were healed in the atonement on the cross?'* Yet despite what we are seeing and feeling, if we are to minister God's healing to others we have to maintain the truth of the word.

When we arrived in San Antonio on the Monday night, neither Dorothy nor I were very good advertisements for healing and wholeness. Bob and Nora cared for us and pampered us until our first meeting with the team from the Order of St Luke on the Wednesday evening. God made the hairs on the back of my neck stand on end that evening, and all my nerves tingle. As I walked into the room at the church, with my body still reeling under the effects of the infection and surgery, a man walked over to me and said, *"I'm Will Bellamy and when you came to this church five years ago I was healed of Parkinson's disease."*

This is Will's story as he wrote it out for me.

What's Shakin'? A true story of healing Parkinson's by prayer

It was one of those days at work that you thought would never end. It was my fiftieth birthday, but all I could do was think about going home, putting my feet up and having a cold beer. When I got there, Donna sang happy birthday in her angelic, off key voice, and said to hurry up because we had somewhere to go for dinner. I tried to beg off nicely but Donna was insistent. I told her that I felt really bad and hoped we could eat quickly so I could fulfill my birthday wish to fall out on my sofa. Donna then broke into tears and had to explain that she had arranged a surprise, and that about twenty or thirty good friends were to be there. I went into shock. I was trapped. The only thing to do was go and pray for deliverance. We pulled up to the restaurant and upon walking into the banquet I discovered that my future bride had really gone to considerable effort and expense. A wonderful party was going on independently from whatever gloom I could generate. The care with which everything was done wore me down, and little by little I was enjoying the party in spite of myself. Toward the end of the evening I was told it was time to open presents. For whatever reason, I was laboring away clumsily, when

I overheard one of my oldest friends ask Donna if I had suffered a stroke. I now knew something was wrong. The very next day I made an appointment to see a neurologist and jotted down a few symptoms to discuss. After watching me walk, make a fist and say the last five presidents backwards, the doctor said, "Parkinson's."

In instant denial I said, "OK, let's run the tests." Doctor said there aren't any beyond this exam and the proof is that we give you the medication and if it works, then you have P.D. I felt that someone had just put a big sandwich board sign on me, which said 'Kick me, I've got P.D.' In a daze I drove home with visions of wheelchairs dancing in my head. I decided to tell Donna immediately, because I had just proposed marriage to her and thought it only fair to give her a chance to back out. To my gratification she said she would stay with me and that we would fight this thing together. She, as a health care professional, had great knowledge of nutrition and pressure point massage therapy. She also knew one of the top neurologists in the city. This neurologist was more careful in his testing and diagnosis but did concur that it most likely was early onset P.D. Donna and I were determined to defeat this condition, and set out on a multipronged attack using every type of weapon available that was logical. I was an avid bicyclist, not adverse to rigid health regimen. So it was with high hopes that we jumped into the fray.

After a year or so, our hopes were beginning to wane. My left hand was constantly jerking, to the extent that my brother once took the telephone receiver away to keep me from clocking myself in the head. I used to be a fairly good guitarist, at one point even touring with Willie Nelson, back in the mid seventies. Now the left hand was a useless claw. Dragging my left foot, my walk had turned into a Frankenstein parody, and with slurred speech many had thought I had turned to the bottle. More medication turned me into a zombie.

I was just about to call the situation hopeless when Donna brought me news of a healing prayer mission up at the Methodist church. There was to be a couple from England, the Vickers, she said; many of the people at the church were excited about it, and would I go? Though intrigued that this main line conservative Methodist church would allow such a thing, I politely declined, saying I had seen some people on TV that looked dubious, and besides I was averse to making a public spectacle. Donna politely said, "You're going."

Things had gotten so bad that an incident of public spectacle was a small price for even long odds of healing. Yet I imagined watching my two heel marks follow us up the sidewalk as a couple of ushers dragged me kicking and screaming into the sanctuary where there would be weirdness.... But, when we arrived, the sanctuary was candlelit with soft lights and quiet music and an air of peace. We were ushered into queues and, as I came closer to the front, I felt as if my heart was beating around in my chest like tennis shoes in a dryer. When I reached the front, a lovely lady grabbed me firmly by the shoulders and asked what I would have Jesus do for me. I said heal my body of Parkinson's. She looked me straight and said, "By the power and the promise of the Lord Jesus Christ you are healed." With those words echoing in my ears, I found myself falling backwards and being caught by my senior pastor, who was as surprised as I was. When I opened my eyes I realized that I was on my back looking up at the vaulted ceiling of the church, ringed by faces looking down at me, praying in some language I could not understand. My confusion was compounded by my inability to get up.

After a long while I got to my feet and was interested to see the sanctuary was like a war zone with people lying about on their backs all over the place. Amazed at this sight, it was a while before I noticed that the trembling had stopped in my left shoulder, arm and hand. At that point people noticed and said, "Look, he's not shaking anymore." There was a chorus of praise from the intercessors and I'm not sure which was the better feeling —being healed or the knowledge that I had most certainly been touched by Christ Jesus.

The trembling did come back, but by then I knew I had something that could touch deeper than medication. So precious, persistent Donna and I joined the Wednesday night prayer team. I was to receive prayer over the next two years, and upon future testing Dr Huey said that I was getting better and what was going on —I was supposed to get worse, not better. When I told him it was the power of prayer he said it must be and to keep it up.

Now, we are eight years free from P.D. I've since seen instant healing, but mine is incremental and needs maintenance over time. I play guitar better than ever, having promised God I would make new music for him. I give constant thanks and praise to the Lord and Father God Jehovah Rapha, the Holy Spirit —and most especially to Randy and Dorothy Vickers. Randy remarked, "Isn't it strange how God always gets funny little people to do his work." That was the first time I've ever rejoiced in being a funny little person. Amen, amen and amen.

Will Bellamy

Cured of coeliac disease

This visit in 2004 turned out to be most interesting in a number of ways. One Wednesday evening Dorothy and I went out to speak and minister at a new church that Scott Heare, a pastor at Alamo Heights, and some of the congregation were planting, about twenty miles out of town. One of the members came up to me and said that she wanted to thank me, because the last time I spoke at Alamo Heights her teenage daughter had been healed of coeliac disease. [Back in 2003 Dorothy and I had been just visiting our friends Nora and Bob but Scott Heare had asked if I would preach on the Sunday morning at the New Heights service, which he led in the Life Centre, as an alternative to the normal Sanctuary service.] It was at this New Heights service that her daughter had attended without her mother. The lady told me that on that Sunday, when her daughter came home from church, she had seen her start to eat something that should certainly have made her ill. When she intervened, the girl said that she had had prayer at the service and had been healed. You can imagine her mother's consternation but, as she said, time had proved it to be true. I was able on that night at Riverside to get the girl to leave the youth group and come and give testimony herself. She told how when she was listening to the talk on that Sunday morning she had felt a sensation in her stomach and knew something was happening. She had then gone forward for prayer at the time for ministry, and just knew she was healed and did not need to worry about what she ate any more. *"Oh," she said, "it is really cool at parties now."*

As I cannot repeat too often, Jesus is the healer; all he has asked us to do is believe in him, preach that the kingdom of heaven is at hand, and he promises that these signs will follow. When we do this, we should expect people to receive. It is the power of his presence, not any gift or power of ourselves. Nor do I expect to know all that he is doing, but it is wonderful when, years later, you start to hear just what he was busy doing at the time.

The Holy Spirit changes churches

On the visit in 2004 I was invited to speak at the Sunday morning services in the Sanctuary rather than at New Heights, and was introduced to his congregation by Pastor David McNitzky.

He said that when Dorothy and I had come to their church some years earlier, the church had been changed. He was referring to the year in which Will Bellamy was healed.

David had invited Dorothy and myself to lead a retreat over the first weekend on inner healing and emotional wholeness. Then morning and evening, Monday through Friday, to teach on various aspects of Jesus' ministry of healing and the gifts of the Holy Spirit. This was mainly for the church prayer team and other members of the congregation who were interested. Finally, on the Sunday evening, we were to lead a healing service in the Sanctuary.

I thought God was amazing to be able to arrange all this and make the weekend and the teaching times virtually full. Apart from that one evening visit, no one knew of us. Randy and Dorothy Vickers are not famous names. God had a great helper, organiser and enthusiast in Nora Scott. Nora had received such blessing, grace and healing from Jesus some years earlier when, through another friend, we had visited with them for an evening, that she wanted everyone else to be able to have at least the same opportunity.

The weekend and the teaching sessions seemed to go very well. However, each time I came to pray for people to be baptised in the Spirit, Scott Heare was missing. All the team received the anointing in power from above, but not Scott. It was this which led eventually to Carolyn praying for Will Bellamy in the way that she did.

We came to the Sunday evening and the time for ministry. To everyone's surprise some 400 people showed up for the service. The prayer team had expected that at the time for ministry all the people would come forward to Dorothy and me to be prayed for. I finished the talk and asked the prayer team to take their places in pairs at the front of the church and invited all who wanted prayer to come forward. Normally in the UK people stay in their seats until they see a prayer team member that has no customers. No sooner had I issued the invitation than all the prayer teams found a long line of clients standing before them. Scott Heare was due to partner Carolyn, but as he was crossing in front of me to reach her I asked him if he had received the Holy Spirit yet. As Scott replied 'no', the Holy Spirit fell on him. I did not touch him; I was not within yards of him. The Holy Spirit fell, and Scott fell, all 6 feet 4 inches or more of him. He lay spreadeagled across the floor in front of the communion table, and was out in the Spirit for a long time.

Carolyn is the person Will refers to in his testimony as a lovely lady. She was standing without a partner; she looked up, and saw Will in front of her starting to fall under the power of the Holy Spirit. She had never before experienced anyone falling under the power of the Holy Spirit when she was ministering to them, and she had no one to catch him. So she grabbed Will by the shoulders to hold him up, quickly spoke his healing into him, and then let him fall, as the senior pastor, David McNitzky, moved forward to catch him.

I think all the members of the prayer team were amazed at how God worked through them in power that evening, at how the anointing of the Holy Spirit fell on people as they prayed. We will never know all the wonderful experiences and healings that Jesus ministered into peoples' lives that night. This was truly a picture of the church, the body of Christ, in the anointing of the Holy Spirit, carrying out his commission to preach the kingdom and heal the sick.

On the Monday morning, at a debriefing session with the staff, Bob Scott stood up and drew a line on the blackboard. Bob said that there came a time in the life of the church when they reached a line and had to decide whether or not they were willing or wanted to cross it. Scott spoke out to say, "Bob, last night we went way over that line and there is no going back."

Healed of coeliac disease and a pituitary disorder
Joan came to Beggars Roost and then wrote to us:
Dear Dorothy and Randy,

Just a note as you came to my mind today —for whenever I thank God for my healing I remember you both and Annie. Perhaps you remember me? (Coeliac disease and a pituitary disorder.) I came on Thursdays at the end of April and the beginning of May 1997, and was instantly restored to health following a 'word of knowledge' to Dorothy. I also met you at the Blyth Coffee Club at the end of May, where you got me up to give testimony.

The good health continues and I have been asked to give testimony many times. Sometimes this has been in front of large gatherings, including ministers and even a former President of the Methodist

Conference. I find that people are always thrilled to hear what happened to me, and the change in my health is so obvious that no-one who knows me can be sceptical.

I have returned to almost full time work as a teacher, and also to my preaching and tutoring work on the Methodist circuit. Peter and I do hope to get across to Stocksfield again and look forward to worship there.

Thank you again for your ministry. God bless you and all the team.

With love, Joan Short

In May 2005 Joan's husband sent me an email with her permission to use her story. He said that she returned to work the next day after her healing and has now accepted a contract to continue working past the age of sixty.

Helen came to Beggars Roost

Helen first wrote to me because she had met with a couple who lived near her, and she had heard the story of how the husband had been healed from Parkinson's disease, through the healing Centre, directly from them. She wanted to come over to discuss the possibility of having prayer to heal the rheumatoid arthritis she had had for 22 years. She wrote that she had had lots of prayer from various groups but had not felt any benefit. I invited her to join us at a Thursday night healing service. Following her visit she sent a second letter:

Dear Rev. Vickers,

It was so good to meet you and your ministry team when I visited you on 6th April 2000. I thought that you might like to know what's been happening to me! First of all, driving back that night my hands were incredibly hot and tingling. I could hardly keep hold of the steering wheel. Every day since, the strength has improved, and I can hold a mug with one hand not two. Secondly, the lump behind my right knee has gone. Praise God for these things and I look forward to more physical healing. I'm living in my healing as you taught.

In 2005, when Helen wrote to give me permission to use her name in this book, she said that the consultant had recently confirmed that she was still in remission from the rheumatoid arthritis. She also added, *My healing I feel has also been from the inside. All the bitterness, resentment and loneliness has gone. I live in my healing and rejoice in being the person God created me to be.*

The healing from Parkinson's disease, to which she referred
A couple contacted me because they had heard of the Centre from others. The husband had been crippled with Parkinson's disease for years, and they wanted to come over and see me. They did come and, although they went home encouraged, there did not appear to be any significant release. However, some time later, a member of their church invited us to bring the team and hold a healing service in their village church on a Sunday. It was a very good evening and I know the Lord was healing in many ways. Early in the service, I prayed with the couple —and, again, no apparent advancement. I then carried on with the service, but Joan from our team was led to stay at the back of the church with him as he sat in his wheelchair. She was convinced that his healing was there if she just hung in beside him in prayer. This is what Paul meant when he referred to gifts of healing. As I was talking I became aware that the man was up out of his wheelchair, and was walking down the aisle. By the end of the evening he seemed completely free. The lady who organised the meeting wrote and told me that on the next day he had walked down his garden, which was quite steep, all on his own, so that he could spend time in his garden shed. This was something he had not been able to do for ages. Quite a while afterwards, his wife wrote and apologised that she had taken so long to communicate but they had been working through a lot of things. This included side effects of withdrawal from the medicines which he had been taking, as the body was cleared of the toxins. I heard nothing more until three or four years later, when the lady who had moved to their village heard the story of his remarkable healing and wanted some for herself. God is so good.

Dorothy and I praise God for these and so many other testimonies. With God all things are possible. If there is anything in this book which has encouraged you, please give all the glory to God.

The work of The Northumbrian Centre of Prayer for Christian Healing is undergirded by the power of prayer. Each month, a large team of home intercessors, who have committed to pray daily, receive a prayer letter, a copy of the Centre diary, and the names and situations of four or five people for whom prayer has been requested. If you are being called to intercessory prayer, please contact us.